ISBN: 978-0-9788603-5-6

Have Stethoscope, Will Travel. Staff Care's Guide to Locum Tenens

First printing – September 2009

Printed in the United States of America

Practice Support Resources, Inc., Publisher

Additional copies of this book may be ordered by calling 1-800-967-7790 or visiting www.PracticeSupport.com.

 This book is for informational purposes only. It is not intended to constitute legal or financial advice. If legal, financial or other professional advice is required, the services of a competent professional should be sought.

HAVE STETHOSCOPE, WILL TRAVEL.

STAFF CARE'S GUIDE TO LOCUM TENENS

By Timothy Boes, Aaron Ray and Phillip Miller

Staff Care is an AMN Healthcare Company.

5001 Statesman Drive
Irving, Texas 75063

800-685-2272
469-524-1473

StaffCare.com
AMNHealthcare.com

Acknowledgements}

The authors would like to thank Kurt Mosley, Vice President of Business Development for Staff Care; Kim Anderson, Director of Administrative Operations; and Courtney Stiles, Licensing Manager, for their invaluable assistance in providing information for this book.

Special thanks also to Steve Schaumburg, Director of Marketing & Brand Management, who formatted the book, and to Ela Whitten, Senior Graphic Designer, who created the jacket design.

In addition, we would like to thank the thousands of physicians and other healthcare professionals we have worked with over the years who have devoted their energy and skills to providing outstanding care to their patients.

ABOUT THE AUTHORS

Timothy Boes

Timothy Boes is President of Staff Care, the nation's leading locum tenens physician staffing firm and an AMN Healthcare Company. AMN Healthcare is the largest healthcare staffing company in the United States. Mr. Boes has more than 28 years of healthcare industry experience in both the private and public sectors. Prior to joining Staff Care, Mr. Boes spent more than 11 years with Cardinal Health, where he served as a regional vice president, group vice president of Integrated Solutions and as the national vice president of sales for their Pharmaceutical Distribution company. In that role, he was responsible for the sales and marketing functions of the hospital segment of Cardinal Health's largest division. As president of Staff Care, Mr. Boes is responsible for setting the strategic direction of the company, setting its budgetary goals and managing daily operations. Mr. Boes received his degree in Healthcare Administration from Ithaca College and resides with his family in Dallas, Texas.

Aaron Ray

Aaron Ray is Senior Vice President of Staff Care and has direct leadership responsibilities for all production and sales functions within the company. Mr. Ray has more than 10 years of experience with Staff Care. Positions held by Mr. Ray at Staff Care include director of recruiting, regional vice president and divisional vice president for the company's Primary Care Division. Mr. Ray is one of the leading authorities on the locum tenens staffing industry in the United States, with expertise in all areas of locum tenens contracting, planning and operations. Mr. Ray graduated from Oklahoma State University and lives with his wife in Dallas, Texas.

Phillip Miller

Phillip Miller is Vice President of Communications for Staff Care and Merritt Hawkins & Associates, AMN Healthcare companies. Mr. Miller has been with Staff Care since the company's inception in 1992 and has more than 20 years of corporate communications and public relations experience. Mr. Miller is author or co-author of more than 400 articles on healthcare staffing and other topics, and also is co-author of the books *Will the Last Physician in America Please Turn Off the Lights? A Look at America's Looming Doctor Shortage; Merritt Hawkins & Associates Guide to Physician Recruiting;* and *Physicians: In Their Own Words.* Mr. Miller graduated from the University of Texas at Austin and lives with his family in Dallas, Texas.

Contents}

Foreword} Who Was that Masked Man? i

Chapter 1} Physicians: An Endangered Species? 1

Chapter 2} Strategic Uses of Locum Tenens 9

Chapter 3} Costs/Benefits 16

Chapter 4} Who's Hitting the Road? 21

Chapter 5} A Locum Tenens FAQ for Physicians 25

Chapter 6} Orientation and the Assignment 36

Chapter 7} Meet the "Country Doctors of the Year" 44

Chapter 8} Tales from the Road 52

Chapter 9} The Licensing Process 58

Chapter 10} Hospital Privileging 76

Chapter 11} Covering Your Tail 80

Addendum} Staff Care's 2009 Review of Temporary Physician Staffing Trends 83

FOREWORD}

WHO WAS THAT MASKED MAN?

"Hi, ho Silver away!"
~ THE LONE RANGER

It's a plot device used by countless movies and TV shows. A stranger rides into town, clears out the bad guys, then rides off into the sunset before anyone can so much as say "thank you."

Most of us don't get to fulfill this "Lone Ranger" fantasy in our daily lives. As a rule, we are tied to the same places and the same faces every day. Not so for the growing number of physicians who work on a temporary basis traveling from one community to another.

Known as "locum tenens," a Latin phrase meaning (more or less) "holding a place," temporary doctors see millions of patients each year and provide services everywhere from top 10 metropolitan hospitals to isolated Indian Health System clinics. They are part of a broader trend in healthcare toward a mobile workforce composed of tens of thousands of physicians, nurses and allied healthcare professionals who work temporary assignments in a wide variety of practice settings and geographic locations.

Locum tenens doctors arrive in a new town, deal with the "bad guys" (flu, broken bones, weakened hearts—even brain tumors) and are then on to their next assignment. For physicians who enjoy variety and travel, locum tenens provides an enviable work style, whether practiced only a couple of weekends a year on a "moonlighting" basis or practiced full-time year round.

In this book we look at why an increasing number of physicians are choosing to work as "locums" and why hospitals, medical groups and other healthcare facilities use temporary doctors. We also examine what doctors need to know about locum tenens practice and what healthcare facilities need to know about working with temporary doctors.

While the focus is on practical matters such as logistics, licensure, malpractice and hospital privileging, we have also included some "tales from the road"—stories by locum tenens doctors about some of their more dramatic or memorable assignments. One chapter we point to with particular pride concerns Country Doctor of the Year Award. In this chapter you will meet some of the most dedicated and revered doctors in America.

Let's begin, however, by discussing where locum tenens physicians fit into the overall healthcare staffing puzzle. Why is there a need for doctors who travel from one assignment to another? Why do healthcare facilities choose to work with these doctors?

And are temporary doctors likely to be a fixture in healthcare or is locum tenens merely a fad that is destined to fade?

1}

PHYSICIANS … AN ENDANGERED SPECIES?

> *"Don't it always seem to go that you don't know what you've got 'til it's gone?"*
> ~ **Joni Mitchell**

Most people, it is safe to say, don't think about doctors until they need one. In our society, the presence of physicians is a given. The same could be said about policemen, accountants, lawyers, bakers, business executives, bankers and those in a variety of other occupations.

The reality, however, is that physicians are not simply part of the professional landscape to be accessed where and when they are needed. They are the end product of a rigorous and expensive selection and training process. The doctor one sees is the tip of the iceberg that is medical education, training and practice. If what lies beneath the surface of the water melts away, the tip also will be in jeopardy.

That is the point we are reaching today. The supply of physicians has become so tenuous that even those with healthcare insurance are having a hard time accessing physicians. Consider the study that appeared in an October 2008 issue of the *Journal of the American Medical Association* (JAMA). The article examined overcrowding in the nation's hospital emergency departments (EDs) and concluded that ED overcrowding is not being driven by uninsured patients seeking treatment for non-urgent problems, as has been popularly believed for years. The study indicates that while 17 percent of the population lacks health insurance, uninsured patients account for only 10 to 15 percent of ED visits. The study further shows that uninsured patients tend to put off treatment until the last moment, so that when they do come to the ED they are genuinely in need of care.

The real driver of hospital ED overcrowding, according to the study, is insured patients who may not be able to access physicians in a timely manner. As Manya Newton, M.D., lead author of the study, put it in an interview with Newsweek.com (10/22/08):

"There are fewer primary care doctors now, so it's hard to get appointments. If you call your doctor's office and say, 'I'm super-sick and coughing up green stuff,' and they say, 'we'll see you three weeks from Tuesday,' you might think you need to go to the emergency room instead. And you might be right."

The fact is that America, for all its wealth and technology, is running out of doctors. How could a nation with thousands of hospitals and countless pieces of highly sophisticated medical equipment be short of the people needed to man those hospitals and operate that equipment?

The simple answer is that demand for doctors exceeds supply. The full answer is a little more complicated and would take a separate book to address. Executives with our affiliate company, Merritt Hawkins & Associates, have written this book which is titled *Will the Last Physician in America Please Turn Off the Lights? A Look at America's Looming Physician Shortage.* It is available through our publisher, Practice Support Resources (www.practicesupport.com), for those who would like a more complete explanation of the physician shortage.

Here we'll only supply a cursory discussion of the shortage, with a focus on how locum tenens fits into the overall picture. Our goal is to show that doctors are not a resource to be taken for granted, but are, in fact, an endangered species that, at least in some specialties, may be on the road to extinction.

DOCTORS – WHO NEEDS 'EM?

Demand for doctors, like demand for just about anything else, does not remain static. It ebbs and flows, though in the case of doctors in the United States, demand rises consistently over time. Richard Cooper, M.D., a nationally noted expert on physician supply and demand trends, observes that demand for physicians rises parallel to economic growth. "Ultimately it is the capacity of a society to purchase healthcare," Dr. Cooper writes, "that determines how many services will be used." *(Annals of Surgery,* October 2007*)*

Though the U.S. economy goes through fits and starts (and is in a down period as we write this), prosperity in this country—which includes the ability to purchase physician services—historically has always increased over time.

In short, Americans have money and one of the things we spend it on (to the tune of several trillion dollars a year) is healthcare. In fact, U.S. healthcare spending, if considered by itself as an "economy," would be the fourth-largest economy in the world.

There are other key factors, however, driving demand for doctors besides the economy. One is population growth. The U.S. Census Bureau projects that America will add 50 million people to its population between 2000 and 2020. That is roughly equivalent to absorbing the population of England within 20 years. According to the U.S. Bureau of Health Professions (BHP), Americans visit physicians an average of three times per person per year, leading to the equation below:

50,000,000 new population x 3 annual visits = 150,000,000 new visits

That is 150 million more doctor visits that will need to be handled in a two-decade period based on population growth alone. This equation assumes that the number of physician visits Americans generate per capita will remain fixed at three, which is unlikely to be the case. In recent years, the per capita number of patient visits has grown steadily, according to the BHP.

This trend is likely to continue since older people visit physicians more times per capita than do younger people, as the table below indicates:

AVERAGE PHYSICIAN VISITS BY AGE

Age	Doctor Visits per Year
60 and older	6.0
46-65	5.4
36-45	3.5
25-35	2.2
16-24	1.5
0-15	2.0
Overall average	3.0

Source: National Ambulatory Medical Care Survey

In 2011, the first of some 80 million baby boomers will begin turning 65. This surge of Medicare-eligible seniors will create a corresponding spike in demand for doctors. The state of Florida provides a snapshot of what the future holds. According to the U.S. Census Bureau, by 2030 the entire country will be, on average, as old as Florida is now.

If current trends continue, not only will we be older on average in coming years, we will be fatter. Obesity increased 60 percent from 1991 to 2000 and about one-third of adults over 20 (about 72 million Americans) are obese, according to the Centers for Disease Control (CDC). Obesity is the root of many medical problems and, along with a variety of other lifestyle and societal conditions, is likely to boost demand for doctors in the future.

Another reason demand for doctors is increasing is that there is so much more physicians can do today than they could in the past. Doctors were once limited to advising patients to "take two aspirin and call me in the morning." Today, there is an endless battery of tests, procedures and pharmaceutical treatments that doctors can prescribe. Whether it's bariatric surgery or non-invasive procedures such as virtual colonoscopies, patients want the latest and greatest care available. It takes a lot of physicians in a variety of medical specialties to provide that care.

An "x factor" that may significantly affect demand for physicians is healthcare reform. It can be assumed that if more people had access to healthcare coverage, more people would seek access to care. The consulting firm The Lewin Group determined that a universal healthcare system would create the need for 35,000 more physicians (Forbes.com, 3/26/07). Even without reform, however, it can be confidently predicted that demand for healthcare services is going nowhere but up.

IS THERE A DOCTOR IN THE HOUSE?

Given a rising population and the other factors noted above, this would seem to be a good time to start training considerably more doctors. We are not doing so, however. In fact, the *net* number of physicians in the United States is decreasing at the precise time when demand for physicians is spiraling upward.

There are several reasons for this. One is that the number of physicians coming out of residency training has remained virtually flat at about 24,000 per year over the last 25 years. Much of doctor training that takes place in the nation's teaching hospitals is funded through Medicare. Funding that Medicare provides to train doctors was capped in 1997 through the Balanced Budget Act because it was thought at that time that the U.S. had too many physicians. Unless the cap is removed, it is unlikely that the number of physicians trained in the U.S. will increase significantly.

There are more than 100,000 medical residents in training in the U.S. today, about one-quarter of whom are graduates of international medical schools. Residents represent an important part of the overall physician workforce and they often treat uninsured, Medicare and Medicaid patients at the nation's mostly urban teaching hospitals. In the past, it was common for residents to work 100 hours a week. In 2002, a law was passed to limit resident working hours to 80 per week—a positive step in terms of quality of care but one which diminishes overall physician supply. Put in concrete terms, the reduction in resident hours eliminates some 20,000 resident full-time-equivalents (FTEs) from the workforce.

Another factor suppressing the net supply of physicians is the feminization of medicine. Medicine was once an almost exclusively male profession. Women interested in providing healthcare usually became nurses while men became doctors. That has changed. More than 50 percent of all medical school entrants today are women and women now dominate the ranks of many residency programs, particularly in primary care. This is another positive step in terms of patient care, but one which greatly constrains physician supply because, on average, female physicians work 20 percent fewer hours than do male physicians (*Annals of Medicine,* 11/2/02*)*. Many female physicians enter medicine during their peak child-rearing years and it typically is their dual role as physicians and mothers that causes them to work fewer hours than male physicians.

Male or female, Generation X and Y physicians often put a higher premium on "quality of life" than do baby boomer doctors. This means they prefer practices that offer regular hours, vacation time and minimal on-call duties so they can spend more time with their spouses and families. The practice styles of younger physicians may lead to a better adjusted workforce, which can in turn have positive quality of care implications. However, the more lifestyle-conscious practice style of many younger doctors today means that one new physician entering the workforce may not replace an older doctor leaving it.

Like the general population, physicians are aging. More than one-third of doctors in the U.S. today are 55 years of age or older. The consulting firm MGT of America projects that by 2016 the number of physicians leaving the field will exceed the number of U.S.-trained physicians entering it. In effect, more water will be flowing out of the tub than will be added and a lot more people will want to take a bath.

As a result, there will be an acute shortage of physicians in the next 10 to 15 years. Dr. Cooper projects a deficit of some 200,000 doctors by the year 2025. The Association of American Medical Colleges and the Council on Graduate Medical Education projections are less dire—a doctor deficit in the 90,000 range by 2020—but are nevertheless sobering. Indeed, former American Medical Association (AMA) president J. Edward Hill has written that the coming physician shortage is "no less ominous" a threat to the nation's health than a pandemic (*American Medical News,* 2/20/06*)*.

By all indications, the shortage will be particularly acute in primary care. Primary care doctors—general internists, family physicians and pediatricians—are paid significantly less than most surgical and diagnostic specialists and generally enjoy a less controllable lifestyle. As a result, primary care has become one of those jobs that few Americans find attractive. More than 50 percent of first-year family practice medical residents in 2007 were international medical graduates, as were more than 40 percent of first-year internal medicine residents. In a sign of what the future holds, a September 2008 article in JAMA indicated that only 2 percent of medical students plan to become general internists. Unless steps are taken to address pay and practice style issues, primary care physicians may go the way of the dinosaur.

SEEKING ALTERNATIVES

There is another trend to be considered, which forms part of the submerged iceberg alluded to earlier that many people don't see. Doctors as a whole are not a happy group. Many are disillusioned—not with patient care but with the overall medical practice environment, which is rife with bureaucracy, reimbursement hassles, malpractice concerns and stress.

In a survey that included responses from some 12,000 physicians conducted by Merritt Hawkins & Associates for the Physicians' Foundation, a non-profit, grant-making organization composed of physician and medical society leaders, 78 percent of doctors surveyed said medicine has become less satisfying over the past five years. Twenty-seven percent said they would not choose medicine as a career if they had it to do over again and 60 percent said they would not recommend medicine as a career to young people.

Physician dissatisfaction has reached a point where many doctors are seeking alternatives to traditional independent practice. When asked what they plan to do in the next one to three years, 11 percent of physicians surveyed said they planned to retire, more than 20 percent said they plan to cut back on the number of patients they see, 10 percent said they plan to work part-time, 10 percent said they will seek jobs outside of medicine, seven percent said they will open concierge practices and *7.5 percent said they will work locum tenens.*

WHERE LOCUM TENENS FITS

Though it has taken us some time to work around to the topic of locum tenens, we have finally hit on it. There is a growing physician shortage at a time when many doctors are looking to escape what they view as an increasingly irksome practice environment. Locum tenens is an emerging practice style that offers an enticing alternative to the traditional private practice option.

Working as a locum tenens offers physicians a variety of attractions. As independent contractors, they are paid by whichever locum tenens staffing firms they choose to partner with—they do not have to submit any bills to third-party payers or worry about collections. They also do not have to manage an office or worry about personnel issues, rent, equipment, patient records or related administrative matters. Malpractice insurance, transportation and housing needed when on a locum tenens assignment are all provided by the staffing agency.

For a growing number of doctors, locum tenens offers a way to avoid the "business of medicine" while still doing what they were trained to do and what they love to do—treat patients. Locum tenens represents a part of the segmentation of the physician workforce that was once a widely homogenous group of office-based doctors running their own small businesses. Today, physician practice styles are considerably more varied. Many doctors work as hospital employees (sometimes as "hospitalists"), some work part-time, others work shift schedules, some have opened "boutique" or "concierge" practices and still others work on a locum tenens basis.

Hospitals, medical groups, government facilities and other organizations seeking physicians need to adapt to ongoing changes and ensure that their staffing plans accommodate these shifting medical practice patterns. They are doing so by employing physicians, creating latitude for part-time doctors or those who want to share their practices, providing flexible vacation time and shift schedules, providing teleradiology coverage, creating hospitalist programs and incorporating locum tenens physicians into their strategic staffing plans.

In Staff Care's 2009 Review of Temporary Physician Staffing Trends we asked hospital and medical group administrators about their use of locum tenens:

Have you used locum tenens physicians to supplement your existing staff in the last 12 months?

Yes 72%
No 28%

In a typical month, how many locum tenens physicians do you use?

None	37%
1-3	20%

4-6	37%
7 or more	6%

Source: Staff Care 2009 Review of Temporary Physician Staffing Trends

As the numbers above show, about three-quarters of hospitals and medical groups indicated they have recently used locum tenens physicians, while 63 percent said they typically use at least one locum tenens physician per month.

In a time of physician shortages, locum tenens helps bolster overall physician supply by keeping older physicians "in the game" when they otherwise might have retired. It also gives younger physicians who may need flexible schedules an opportunity to be active in the workforce, seeing patients rather than staying home full-time. For physicians in mid-career, locum tenens can serve as a bridge from one opportunity to another, allowing them to be productive while transitioning to a new practice.

It is important to consider that the *net supply* of physicians is shrinking. Retirement, changing practice styles, the cap on resident hours and the growing number of female physicians all tend to reduce the number of full-time equivalent doctors. One exception is locum tenens, where the number of available physicians is actually increasing.

How can hospitals, physician practices and other healthcare organizations best utilize the resources represented by this growing segment of the physician workforce? That is the subject of Chapter Two.

2}

THE STRATEGIC USES OF LOCUM TENENS

> *"If all you have is a hammer, everything looks like a nail."*
>
> ~ **Bernard Baruch**

The use of locum tenens physicians to replace clinicians who have either permanently or temporarily absented themselves from their practices has a long history. The locum tenens staffing industry, however, did not form until the 1970s when the first agencies were established to provide temporary physicians to health facilities in medically underserved areas. Locum tenens physicians initially were used by hospitals and medical groups primarily to provide coverage for doctors on vacation or those pursuing continuing medical education (CME).

At first, physicians working on a locum tenens basis were not always judged favorably by their peers or by healthcare administrators. The perception at the time (and sometimes the reality) was that locum tenens physicians were compromised in some way and so could not maintain permanent, full-time practices. There were only a handful of physicians working on a locum tenens basis at that time.

Locum tenens took a great leap forward in the mid-1990s, when the advent of managed care put a premium on primary care "gatekeeper" physicians. There was a virtual feeding frenzy in the industry in which hospitals and medical groups were feverishly attempting to create networks of physician gatekeepers who would control patient entry into the healthcare system. If permanent primary care physicians could not be found immediately, many medical groups and hospitals turned to locum tenens doctors to "hold a place" until permanent physicians could be recruited.

The gatekeeper system ultimately fizzled in most parts of the country (taking many physician practice management firms with it) and demand for primary care physicians significantly abated. However, another trend developed which kept demand for locum tenens rising. Enhanced medical technology, population growth and population aging created a shortage of specialist physicians that began in the mid-1990s and has continued ever since. The specialist shortage is what drove the use of locum tenens doctors steadily upward during the late 1990s and for much of the current decade.

Today, the physician staffing market is going through yet another cycle. While specialist physicians remain in demand, primary care doctors have returned to the top of the wish list of many hospital and medical group administrators. While demand for primary care doctors in the 1990s was to some extent artificially induced by managed care, demand today is more patient driven. As the population has increased and aged and as fewer physicians choose to specialize in primary care, there is a real rather than an artificially induced shortage of primary care physicians.

Recent demand trends in the locum tenens staffing market are illustrated by Staff Care's annual Review of Temporary Physician Staffing Trends, which tracks the types of physicians most requested by our clients (results of the 2008 study are included at the end of this book). The table below compares the types of physicians our clients requested by specialty over the last several calendar years.

ANNUAL LOCUM TENENS MIX OF "DAYS REQUESTED" BY SPECIALTY

	2004 (%)	2006 (%)	2007 (%)	2008 (%)
Anesthesiology/CRNA	31	22	20	20
Behavioral Health	29	17	18	16
Primary Care	20	41	42	43
Radiology	15	12	12	11
Surgery	5	8	8	8
Dentistry	0	0	2	3

Source: Staff Care 2009 and 2005 Review of Temporary Physician Staffing Trends

The shift in demand toward primary care physicians over a three-year period is readily apparent in this table. What is less apparent is that demand for most other specialties also remains strong, as Staff Care's overall number of temporary days requested significantly increased from 2004 to 2008. Just as in permanent physician placement, the increase in demand for primary care doctors has not signaled a decrease in demand for other specialties. We are now in an era where demand for both generalist primary care doctors and procedurally and diagnostically oriented specialists is growing.

The rising use of locum tenens doctors is underlined by the dollars that hospitals and medical groups are spending on temporary physician staffing, illustrated in the table below.

SIZE OF THE LOCUM TENENS MARKET BY ANNUAL DOLLARS SPENT (IN BILLIONS)

2004	2005	2006	2007	2008	2009
$1.1	$1.2	$1.4	$1.6	$1.9	$2.1

Source: Staffing Industry Analysts

As these numbers indicate, spending on locum tenens staffing has doubled over a six-year period.

The increasing use of locum tenens is a result not just of physician shortages but of the fact that locum tenens physicians are now widely accepted by physicians, healthcare administrators and patients. Part of this acceptance is a function of the malpractice crisis, which has greatly increased the level of scrutiny to which locum tenens physicians are subjected. In order to reduce malpractice risk, the privileging process for locum tenens physicians has become very rigorous—just as rigorous (and in some cases more so) than the process of privileging newly recruited permanent physicians. As a result, both the quality and the reputation of locum tenens physicians have markedly improved and they are generally viewed as being on par with their permanent counterparts.

The Review of Temporary Physician Staffing Trends referenced above includes interviews with hospital and medical group administrators nationwide who were asked about the skill level of locum tenens providers (see table below):

What is your perception of the general skill level of locum tenens providers?

Excellent	16%
Good	50%
Adequate	33%
Unsatisfactory	19%

Source: Staff Care 2009 Review of Temporary Physician Staffing Trends

These numbers indicate that locum tenens physicians now are considered to be qualified physicians by the great majority of hospital and medical group administrators. Given their growing availability and the generally high-quality services they provide, healthcare executives are finding new uses for temporary doctors.

MULTIPLE USES FOR LOCUM TENENS

As hospitals and medical group managers review their physician recruiting strategies, many are considering how locum tenens physicians can be leveraged as part of a comprehensive medical staff plan.

There are a variety of ways in which locum tenens doctors can play a complementary role in physician staff planning. These include:

Vacation, maternity leave, medical leave and CME. The traditional use of locum tenens to provide coverage for temporarily absent physicians has not diminished in recent years and has, in fact, increased due to reasons referenced earlier. Many younger physicians are seeking practices that offer generous vacation time, regular hours and favorable coverage schedules. In addition, the number of female physicians has increased dramatically in recent years and many female physicians require time off because of their dual roles as professionals and home makers. The number of locum tenens "physician days" needed to cover vacation time is running into the millions per year. Some hospitals and medical groups are inclined to simply work their physicians harder or influence their doctors away from taking their allotted vacation time. Others use locum tenens providers to ensure that physicians are able to take vacations as promised and to prevent physician burn out. This serves as both a recruiting tool, helping some hospitals and groups achieve a reputation for being "physician-friendly," and as a retention tool during a time when physician turnover is particularly hard to address.

Placeholder while a permanent search is ongoing. The physician shortage has left many hospitals, medical groups and other facilities understaffed. A growing number of facilities are using locum tenens doctors to maintain services and revenue until permanent candidates can be recruited. In its 2008 Review of Temporary Physician Staffing Trends, Staff Care asked hospital and medical group administrators why they use locum tenens physicians. More administrators (65 percent) cited "to hold a place until permanent staff is recruited" than any other factor.

Physician retirement or disability. More than one-third of physicians in the U.S. today are 55 years of age or older and abrupt physician retirements are not uncommon. When an established physician suddenly turns in his or her stethoscope, locum tenens physicians can maintain continuity of care until the practice can reorganize and adjust. The same is true in cases of physician disability.

Test-marketing new service lines. Many hospitals or large medical groups wish to experiment with new services but hesitate to recruit new physicians full-time in case a viable market does not exist. Some hospitals and groups use locum tenens physicians to gauge patient receptiveness to new services and then make a more informed decision regarding whether or not to add the service. An example is a Staff Care client that test-marketed the viability of establishing a women's center by using a locum tenens obstetrician/gynecologist, anesthesiologist and mammographer to determine the potential case load. This test clearly justified recruiting full-time clinicians and putting them on the payroll. In a variation of this scenario, a client built a new surgery center without first establishing adequate volume and had hired three permanent clinicians without enough cases to make the center profitable. The client released these clinicians to do locum tenens work until it could build adequate volume for the surgery center. The clinicians were able to maintain their income and the client was not burdened with paying their salaries until sufficient volume was established.

Maintain trauma level status. In order to maintain their trauma level status, hospitals must have certain types of physicians continuously on-call. Locum tenens physicians can provide this coverage when local doctors are either unavailable or unwilling to be on-call. Typically, this means providing coverage at night and on weekends.

Expanding into new geographic market areas. Hospitals seeking to establish satellite clinics may not wish to gamble by recruiting a permanent physician to set up practice in a new location. Instead, they may staff the clinic with one or more locum tenens physicians to establish a foothold in the area. If the practice proves viable, they then can recruit a permanent doctor.

Enhance permanent physician recruiting efforts. Hospitals and medical groups can use locum tenens physicians to bolster their permanent physician recruiting efforts. A locum tenens physician can build a patient base so that when a permanent physician joins the community he or she can hit the ground running. In addition, a locum tenens physician with a thriving patient load demonstrates clearly to permanent recruitment candidates that a sound practice really exists. It is not unusual for locum tenens physicians to see the advantages of working for a particular hospital or group and to join the staff full-time.

Prevent patient defections. Healthcare today is becoming more consumer driven and "customer service" has become a greater priority. During flu season or peak usage periods, locum tenens physicians can handle patient overflow and forestall patients who are impatient with lengthy doctor appointment times from seeking care elsewhere.

Secure larger managed care accounts. Hospitals and medical groups seeking large managed care accounts often are reluctant or unable to recruit a significant number of permanent physicians until the account has been secured. However, they cannot secure such accounts until they can demonstrate they have the staff to service the account. By working with a pool of locum tenens physicians, they can demonstrate to the managed care organization that they have the necessary manpower and be sure of the account before they recruit permanent physicians.

Hospital expansion. As hospitals expand, they often allow medical groups to bid on hospital-based services such as radiology or anesthesiology. Groups that may not have the current manpower to handle the hospital's increased volumes can supplement their staffs with locum tenens physicians and remain competitive in the bidding process.

Military duty/deployment. Current military commitments abroad have depleted the supply of physicians in some areas as physician reservists are called up for duty. Locum tenens physicians are being used in many communities to maintain services until reservists can return to their civilian practices. In addition, locum tenens doctors are being used by military bases to maintain services when military physicians are deployed overseas.

Emergencies/natural disasters. In the aftermath of Hurricane Katrina, Staff Care and other locum tenens firms filled many requests for temporary physicians to supply services required because of the disaster.

Maintain revenue. Hospitals and groups considering locum tenens physicians must take a close look at the potential return on investment. While locum tenens physicians are a cost, this cost must be weighed against the revenue locum tenens physicians generate. Locum tenens physicians often more than pay for themselves by maintaining revenues for the hospital or group (see Chapter Three).

Temp-to-permanent. There are some cases in which the locum tenens assignment becomes a "working interview" for the doctor, who may be offered a permanent position by the facility which thereby receives both a short-term and a long-term benefit.

Continuity of care. Last, but not least, quality of care is largely dependent on continuity. Locum tenens physicians can maintain continuity of care for patients when current physician manpower levels are insufficient.

Indeed, even though locum tenens is considered "interim" coverage, some medical groups and hospitals are modifying their staffing models to include an ongoing "float pool" of locum tenens providers. This increases the stability of the hospital department or group as a whole. With a "floater" to provide coverage, the permanent staff can work structured hours, schedule their vacations and enjoy a better work-life balance, which increases physician retention. Staff Care has had locum tenens physicians and CRNAs stay on assignments for more than three years as a locum tenens under this "float pool" model in which locum tenens doctors act as a "reserve unit" capable of filling in on short notice in a variety of scenarios.

By using locum tenens physicians strategically, healthcare facilities and medical practices are better positioned to respond proactively to a changing medical practice environment in which there are a variety of ways to meet staffing needs. Because there is more to work with than a hammer, not everything "looks like a nail."

3}

COSTS/BENEFITS

"A cynic is a man who knows the price of everything but the value of nothing."
~ **Oscar Wilde**

Physicians often put in 12 years or more of costly collegiate and postgraduate training before they can be certified in their respective specialties. They are capable of doing extraordinary things, from diagnosing rare diseases to performing brain surgery and heart replacements. Given their in-depth training and extraordinary skills, it is not surprising that physician services entail a cost, even though under our system of third-party payers, many patients think they are getting to see a doctor for next to nothing.

Locum tenens physicians are generally paid on an hourly or daily basis, with bonuses available for working overtime, nights or weekends. These rates vary based on the supply, demand and other market conditions prevailing in particular specialties. As we write this, daily rates for primary care physicians are rising as the demand for these doctors is growing and the supply is diminishing (see Chapter One). By contrast, daily rates have fallen in radiology, in part because the Deficit Reduction Act of 2007 (DRA) has reduced revenues at some free-standing imaging centers. Falling revenues have caused some radiologists to reduce their vacation time, thereby decreasing the need for locum tenens physicians.

Daily locum tenens rates also are related to what physicians in various specialties typically are paid on a permanent basis. Current reimbursement systems favor physicians who are procedurally oriented over physicians who are consultatively oriented. For that reason, surgical and diagnostic specialists earn more than primary care physicians. The table below indicates average salary offers used to recruit permanent physicians in various specialties as tracked by Merritt Hawkins & Associates:

AVERAGE ANNUAL PHYSICIAN SALARY/INCOME OFFERS BY SPECIALTY

Orthopedic Surgery	$481,000
Radiology	$391,000

Cardiology	$419,000
Urology	$401,000
Gastroenterology	$393,000
Anesthesiology	$344,000
General Surgery	$321,000
Obstetrics/Gynecology	$266,000
Psychiatry	$200,000
General Internal Medicine	$186,000
Family Practice	$184,000
Pediatrics	$171,000

Source: Merritt Hawkins & Associates' 2009 Review of Physician and CRNA Recruiting Incentives

Compare these average annual salary levels for permanent physicians to the current range of daily rates for locum tenens doctors paid by healthcare facilities, physician practices and other organizations to locum tenens agencies. These rates include what agencies pay to physicians and the agencies' fees, and depending on the specialty, can range from less than $1,000 per day to more than $2,000 per day.

The financial and non-financial benefits of using locum tenens doctors must be balanced against these costs. Each year, Staff Care asks hospital and medical group administrators about the benefits of using locum tenens doctors in our Review of Temporary Physician Staffing Trends (see table below).

What are the benefits of using locum tenens physicians?

Continual treatment of patients	36%
Prevent revenue loss	21%
Prevent staff burnout	16%
Immediate availability	20%
Cost	35%
Other	6%

Source: Staff Care 2009 Review of Temporary Physician Staffing Trends

As these numbers suggest, the primary benefit derived from locum tenens physicians is not directly financial in nature. Locum tenens physicians allow for continuity of care and the maintenance of services. The fundamental mission of hospitals and other healthcare organizations is to provide healthcare to their patient populations, a mission they cannot complete without the appropriate number and mix of physicians and other clinicians.

Preventing staff burnout and enhancing retention is another benefit of locum tenens physicians not directly related to finances, though physician retention clearly has a financial impact. Physician defections due to burnout can lead to patient defections which, in turn, have a negative impact on revenue.

In addition to these benefits, locum tenens physicians can provide a direct financial benefit by generating revenue through patient consultations, procedures, tests, prescriptions and hospital admissions. Merritt Hawkins & Associates conducts a survey of hospital chief financial officers to determine how much revenue physicians in various specialties generate on behalf of their affiliated hospitals per year. Annual figures for several specialties are noted in the table below:

AVERAGE ANNUAL INPATIENT/OUTPATIENT REVENUE GENERATED BY PHYSICIANS FOR THEIR AFFILIATED HOSPITALS

Orthopedic Surgery	$2,313,168
Cardiology (Invasive)	$2,662,600
General Surgery	$1,947,934
Internal Medicine	$1,987,253
Family Practice	$1,615,828
Psychiatry	$888,911

Source: Merritt Hawkins & Associates' 2007 Physician Inpatient/Outpatient Revenue Survey

As these numbers suggest, hospitals that have vacancies on their staffs for even a short amount of time can face a significant opportunity cost. The table below shows net revenue lost per month by hospitals that have a vacancy in a variety of specialties. These estimates are based on the Merritt Hawkins & Associates' physician revenue numbers referenced above and assume that physicians generate roughly the same amount of revenue for their hospitals from month to month.

NET REVENUE LOST OVER A PERIOD OF PHYSICIAN VACANCY

Specialty	1 Month	2 Months	3 Months	4 Months	5 Months
Orthopedic Surgery	$192,681	$385,361	$578,042	$770,723	$963,403
Cardiology (Inv.)	$221,883	$443,767	$665,650	$887,533	$1,109,417
General Surgery	$162,328	$324,656	$486,984	$649,311	$811,639
Internal Medicine	$165,604	$331,209	$496,831	$662,418	$828,022

Family Practice	$134,652	$269,305	$403,957	$538,609	$673,262
Psychiatry	$74,076	$148,152	$222,228	$296,304	$370,380

Source: Merritt Hawkins & Associates' 2007 Physician Inpatient/Outpatient Revenue Survey

Another yardstick by which to measure the financial costs/ benefits of locum tenens physicians is provided by the Medical Group Management Association's (MGMA) annual Physician Compensation and Production Survey. This survey tracks the gross daily charges generated by physicians practicing in medical groups (see table below).

AVERAGE GROSS DAILY CHARGES BY PHYSICIANS IN MEDICAL GROUPS

Specialty	Gross Daily Charge
Orthopedic Surgery	$3,292
Cardiology (Invasive)	$7,795
General Surgery	$2,355
Internal Medicine	$1,396
Family Practice	$1,463
Psychiatry	$939

Source: Medical Group Management Association 2007 Physician Compensation and Production Survey

Based on these numbers, a case can be made that the cost of using locum tenens physicians is comparable to the cost of employing a permanent physician.

For example, a family physician paid $180,000 annually costs approximately $720 a day based on five days worked per week during a 50-week year. This excludes signing bonuses, benefits, malpractice premiums, the employer's portion of FICA and continuing medical education expenses—all of which can add more than $60,000 to a physician's total annual compensation package.

The standard per diem rate for a locum tenens family physician, by comparison, is only minimally higher than $720 (including malpractice, travel and housing), roughly equal to the cost of a permanent physician.

Of course, the return on investment with locum tenens is even clearer when the basis of comparison is not a permanent physician, but no physician at all. As indicated above, the MGMA reports that a family physician generates $1,463 in daily charges and Merritt Hawkins & Associates' numbers show that one family physician generates more than $6,400 per day in revenue for his or her affiliated hospital. Rather than an expense, locum tenens physicians can be net revenue generators when they are filling a gap in the medical staff.

There are instances in which the benefits of using locum tenens physicians will be mostly non-financial in nature, pertaining more to continuity of services than to revenue generation. In other cases, using locum tenens physicians will be a break-even proposition from the financial perspective that will prevent revenue loss. However, there are instances in which locum tenens physicians both ensure continuity of services and generate positive revenues.

Regardless of which scenario applies, locum tenens staffing agencies work on a contingent basis, so no expenses are generated until a physician is in place seeing patients and generating revenue.

An additional potential benefit of locum tenens that may offset costs is the fact that, in some cases, healthcare facilities and physician practices are auditioning their facilities and communities for locum tenens doctors. If the doctor likes what he or she sees, it is not unusual for locum tenens physicians to go from temp-to-perm, in which case staffing agencies charge a placement fee. The placement fee may be somewhat higher than would be charged by a physician recruiting company specializing in permanent physician placement. However, the chances of a lasting match may be greater when a locum tenens doctor is recruited to a permanent position, since both the doctor and the facility have gotten to know one another during the locum tenens assignment.

4}

WHO'S HITTING THE ROAD?

> ***"I took the path less traveled by, and that has made all the difference."***
> **~ Robert Frost**

The chances are good that most physician readers of this book know what it means to "hit the wall."

Perhaps it was the latest pre-authorization battle you had to go through with an insurance company or maybe it was the latest rise in your malpractice premiums. Or it could have been the seemingly ceaseless struggle over reimbursement that, like a pebble in a shoe, has become more and more irksome. Turf battles may have figured into it and you may have gotten weary of dealing with personnel issues, administrative hassles and locking horns with the local hospital about ED call, patient records and related issues.

Or maybe none of these things apply. Maybe you are simply at a stage of your career where locum tenens is the right option at the right time.

There are any number of reasons why physicians choose to "hit the road" and try the locum tenens lifestyle. Some of them have to do with the myriad challenges and frustrations presented by traditional medical practice alluded to above and in Chapter One. For some doctors, locum tenens represents an alternative to a traditional private practice model that has become untenable. Other physicians are reaching the end of their careers but still wish to see patients and earn income for at least part of the year.

By contrast, other doctors are just starting out and are curious about different types of medical settings and geographic locations. They use locum tenens to "test drive" various practice styles and areas, "comparison shopping" until they are ready to settle into permanent practice. A fourth type of locum tenens physician is in some sort of transitional phase. They may have a gap between residency and their first permanent practice and will use locum tenens as a way to hone their skills, earn income and see the country before starting their first full-time practice. They may also be in mid-career but have decided to make a change. They use locum tenens to maintain skills and income while determining what they want to do next.

A fifth category of doctor uses locum tenens to earn extra income during free time such as weekends or vacations.

In general, then, physicians who have decided to try locum tenens fall into five categories:

Alternatives:	Physicians seeking a haven from the slings and arrows of the medical practice environment
Sunset seekers:	Highly experienced doctors using locum tenens to cap their careers
Test drivers:	Young physicians curious about what's out there
Transitionals:	Mid-career physicians using locum tenens as a bridge to their next step
Moonlighters:	Physicians using locums to earn extra income during off-hours or extended vacation time

Of course, once they give locum tenens a try, any of these types of doctors are subject to taking the next step—which is becoming a full-time locum tenens physician. There are doctors—and we see their numbers growing—who have made locum tenens their full-time, long-term career option.

In Staff Care's annual Review of Temporary Physician Staffing Trends we survey not just hospital and medical group administrators who use locum tenens doctors, but also doctors who are working or who have worked locum tenens. In our 2009 review, we interviewed 758 locum tenens physicians. The table below shows how they break out in terms of medical practice experience:

How many years have you been in medical practice?

Less than 1 year	2%
1 to 5 years	6%
6 to 10 years	6%
11 to 20 years	19%
21 years or more	67%

Source: Staff Care 2009 Review of Temporary Physician Staffing Trends

These numbers indicate that the majority of locum tenens doctors are more senior physicians who fall into the "sunset seeker" category. However, one third are either "transitionals" or "test drivers." In recent years, we have seen a gradual demographic shift among locum tenens physicians. In the past, locum tenens doctors were predominantly older physicians with two decades or more of experience. Today, locum tenens physicians span the spectrum, from residents with the latest training to veterans who have seen it all.

We also asked physicians in the 2009 review about their locum tenens experience:

How long have you worked as a locum tenens physician?

Less than 1 year	30%
1 to 3 years	26%
More than 3 years	49%

Source: Staff Care 2009 Review of Temporary Physician Staffing Trends

Almost one third of physicians interviewed (30 percent) are new to locum tenens practice. These numbers support our observations in the field, which indicate that the ranks of locum tenens doctors are growing as more doctors give temporary practice a try.

Based on the number of physicians Staff Care matches each year with temporary assignments and on our knowledge of the overall temporary staffing market, we have come up with a rough estimate of the number of physicians who work locum tenens during the course of a given year:

ESTIMATED NUMBER OF DOCTORS WHO WORK LOCUMS DURING THE YEAR

2002	2004	2006	2008
28,000	34,000	36,000	37,000

Source: Staff Care industry estimates

These physicians may have different reasons for practicing locum tenens but they have come to the same conclusion—that locum tenens can address some of their needs at least some of the time. In our review we asked physicians what they like about locum tenens:

What are the benefits of working as a locum tenens physician?

Freedom/flexibility	31%
No politics	19%
Travel	18%
Pay rate	15%
Professional development	9%
A way to find a permanent job	7%

Source: Staff Care 2009 Review of Temporary Physician Staffing Trends

We also asked physicians what they consider to be the downside of working locum tenens:

What are the drawbacks of working as a locum tenens physician?

Away from home	31%
Uncertainty of assignments	25%
Lack of benefits	17%
Quality of assignments	13%
Other	2%

Source: Staff Care 2009 Review of Temporary Physician Staffing Trends

Physicians who embrace variety and are readily adaptable to new places and new ways of doing things are likely to enjoy locum tenens. Those who require structure and are more comfortable with a set daily routine—or who simply must stay at home to meet family or other obligations—may not adjust to the locum tenens life as easily. While staffing agencies provide logistical support, locum tenens physicians are independent contractors who map out their own courses, choosing where and when they want to work.

Physicians who are intrigued by locum tenens usually have a variety of questions about how locum tenens works. We address some of these frequently asked questions in Chapter Five.

5}

A LOCUM TENENS FAQ FOR PHYSICIANS

> *"A journey of a thousand miles begins with a single step."*
>
> ~ LAO-TZU

As noted in the last chapter, a practice style offering freedom and flexibility is attractive to many physicians. But as romantic as the appeal of hitting the road may be, working as a locum tenens physician involves a number of practical matters that are best understood on the front end.

Following are a number of questions doctors typically ask us when considering locum tenens practice.

HOW DO I FIND LOCUM TENENS WORK?

Some physicians contract directly with hospitals, medical groups and other organizations to provide locum tenens services. The great majority, however, work through staffing agencies that represent a number of different clients seeking locum tenens physicians. The agency matches physicians with clients needing locum tenens coverage and handles many or all of the logistical and administrative necessities of being a locum tenens physician.

WHAT ARE THE ADVANTAGES OF DIRECT CONTRACTING?

The principal advantage is that pay rates in direct contracting may be somewhat higher than those offered by agencies. If the doctor contracts with local hospitals, paperwork and logistical issues may be simplified.

WHAT ARE THE ADVANTAGES OF WORKING THROUGH AN AGENCY?

There are several. One is that agencies represent multiple opportunities regionally and/or nationally. Working through agencies, doctors can stay busy and avoid down times between assignments, which can suppress income. They also can enjoy a wide variety of assignments that may vary geographically and in terms of practice style. An agency may match a physician with a large metropolitan teaching hospital one month and a remote Indian Health Service clinic the next. If a physician enjoys a particular style of practice, such as rural medicine, agencies may be able to provide consistent work that conforms to the physician's wants and needs.

In addition, agencies offer a range of support services that can save physicians considerable time and energy.

WHAT TYPE OF SUPPORT SERVICES DO AGENCIES PROVIDE?

Standards and services differ in the industry, but a reputable, full-service locum tenens staffing agency will offer the following:

- Regular assignments
- Detailed knowledge of the practice setting
- Paid malpractice insurance
- Paid travel to assignments
- Paid accommodation
- Credentialing assistance
- Licensure assistance
- Assignment orientation
- Full logistical support

Full logistical support entails ensuring that the physician's assignment goes as smoothly as possible and that all details regarding licensure, credentialing, travel, accommodation, etc. are handled efficiently. A full-service locum tenens agency also will work to ensure that the physician's skills and availability are compatible with what is required by the agency's client.

HOW SHOULD I PICK AN AGENCY?

Visit the company's Web site to gauge their longevity, services, expertise and professionalism. Check to see if they have received endorsements from third parties such as state hospital associations and if they are members of the National Association of Locum Tenens Organizations (NALTO). Ask for references from other doctors in your specialty with whom the agency has worked. Select a full-service agency that offers the support referenced above. Ask how many assignments they have open in your specialty to ensure the firm is large enough to keep you busy. Evaluate the firm on its efficiency in processing paperwork, the care it takes in matching you to assignments appropriately, how it prepares you for the assignment and the extent to which it is available to assist you during the assignment, if necessary.

At some locum tenens agencies, a single staffer is responsible for bringing in clients, recruiting locum tenens physicians and scheduling them on assignments. Others, such as Staff Care, train specialists who focus on one area and sometimes on one or two specialties within that area. For example, Staff Care's Territory Sales Consultants may specialize in marketing the firm's surgical locum tenens staffing services to facilities in the Northeast. Recruiting Consultants may specialize in finding primary care physicians to accept assignments in the Southwest. This allows our personnel to develop relationships and expertise within the specialty and to address the specific needs and nuances of different medical specialties and different regions of the country.

Here are some questions you may ask when evaluating locum tenens companies:

- How long have you been in business?
- What specialties do you represent?
- Do you offer regional and national opportunities?
- What kind of facilities do you represent?
- Do you represent commercial or government contracts or both?
- Do you represent solo or group practices or both?
- What kind of malpractice insurance do you offer and what are your carriers' ratings?
- Will you take care of travel and lodging?
- Will you take care of licensing and privileging?
- What is the size and financial strength of the company?

In our 2009 Review of Temporary Physician Staffing Trends we asked doctors how they choose locum tenens agencies:

How do you select a locum tenens firm?

Location of opportunities	23%
Customer service	22%
Pay rate	16%
Reputation/name recognition	14%
Number of opportunities	16%
Malpractice insurance	10%
Other	1%

Source: Staff Care 2009 Review of Temporary Physician Staffing Trends

As these numbers demonstrate, variety of assignment locations available is the top reason why physicians choose to work with a particular staffing agency, but the customer service provided by the agency rates second, higher than pay.

CAN I WORK WITH MULTIPLE AGENCIES OR DO I HAVE TO CHOOSE JUST ONE?

As you will note throughout this book, locum tenens physicians are independent contractors. As such, you may choose to work with one agency or you may choose to work with a variety of agencies. Staff Care suggests that physicians and facilities investigate several agencies, at least initially, so that they have a basis for comparing service standards.

DO I HAVE TO AGREE TO A CERTAIN NUMBER OF ASSIGNMENTS OR TO PROVIDE A CERTAIN NUMBER OF DAYS WHEN I SIGN WITH A FIRM OR CAN I PICK ASSIGNMENTS "A LA CARTE"?

The number of assignments you take and the number of days you provide are up to you. You do not have to agree to any specific number of assignments or days when working with locum tenens staffing agencies.

DO I HAVE A CHOICE IN SELECTING WHERE I GO?

Yes. As an independent contractor, you can select where and when you wish to practice. You may select from whatever opportunities the agency presents to you and choose which, if any, assignment you want to take. Agencies should not attempt to dictate where and when you work.

ONCE I SELECT AN AGENCY OR AGENCIES, WHAT HAPPENS NEXT?

Your first contact with an agency may be through a recruiter contacting you to determine if you have an interest in locum tenens practice. The recruiter will obtain information about your medical training, licensure and your personal and professional interests. In some cases, the recruiter will contact you about particular opportunities and then coordinate logistics such as licensure, credentialing, travel, etc. Some firms, such as Staff Care, dedicate an Account Representative to each physician. The Account Representative becomes the physician's partner and ensures coordination of all assignments. At Staff Care, the Account Rep works with both our licensing and credentialing departments to make sure physicians have the documents they need for each assignment.

DO I SIGN A CONTRACT?

Yes. All companies offer one and they may vary. Most contracts are somewhat general in nature and stipulate that the physician has granted the agency permission to present his or her name and credentials to facilities seeking locum tenens doctors. The physician also agrees that, if presented with an opportunity by an agency, he or she will not work at that opportunity through any other agency and will not contract directly with the opportunity. When the physician does agree to work at a particular assignment, he or she will receive a confirmation letter from the agency.

WHAT IS IN THE CONFIRMATION LETTER?

The confirmation letter includes the details of the assignment and should be read carefully. These details usually include:

- Compensation. Will it be daily, hourly and will there be separate rates for additional hours or on-call availability?
- Lodging. Does the contract specify whether or not it will be paid?
- Mileage. Will car expenses be reimbursed and under what circumstances?
- Travel. Will travel be paid for?
- Location. What is the exact location of the assignment?
- Length of assignment. What are the exact dates I will be on assignment and what are the shifts?
- Out clauses. Under what circumstances may I decline an assignment or leave it once I have signed the contract?
- Perm fees. If I should decide to accept a permanent position, what sort of placement fee is the locum tenens agency entitled to and who pays for it?
- Non-compete clauses. What is the staffing firm's non-compete clause? The standard in the industry is as follows: If a staffing firm formally introduces a physician by presenting his or her curriculum vitae (CV) and other documents to a particular location, the physician may not work at that location for a

period of two years unless he or she works through the agency that made the formal introduction.

- Malpractice. What type of insurance is provided and who pays for it?

Review the letter with your staffing agency representative and make sure you understand and are comfortable with the terms.

WHAT IS THE APPROPRIATE WAY FOR A LOCUM TENENS COMPANY TO BOOK ME ON AN ASSIGNMENT?

A representative with the firm must get your permission to submit your CV for a specific assignment. You should know the location of the assignment and the name of the facility to which your CV has been submitted. Firms should not be sending out your CV in a "shotgun" manner to anyone they think may have an interest. The firm should update you regarding the review process and let you know where things stand.

HOW LONG IS THE TYPICAL ASSIGNMENT?

Assignments can vary and may last from one day to more than a year. In general, however, assignment lengths break out as follows:

- Weekend call coverage
- One-week vacation coverage
- 4-6 weeks
- 6 months to one year
- Virtually indefinitely (In government facilities, in particular, locum tenens assignments can last for multiple years.)

DO I HAVE TO QUIT MY JOB OR CAN I MOONLIGHT?

It depends on your specialty—moonlighting tends to be more practical for hospital-based physicians such as radiologists and anesthesiologists than for office-based physicians. Standard moonlighting assignments are for nights and weekends, though today locum tenens assignments are shifting to a full-time model.

WHAT IF I AM OFFERED THE SAME JOB BY TWO DIFFERENT STAFFING COMPANIES?

The industry standard is that you should work with whichever firm first presented you to their client with your permission. Some agencies "shop" physician CVs, sending them out without physician permission, and may claim they submitted your information first. However, if they did so without your permission, their claim is not valid.

Locum tenens contracts stipulate that physicians may not work through agencies that presented an opportunity second, even if they did so with the physician's permission, nor may they contract directly with an opportunity once it has been introduced to them by an agency. As independent contractors, of course, locum tenens physicians are not required to go on any assignment, whether it was presented first, second or in any other order. However, they are required *not* to accept opportunities unless they work through the agency which first introduced the opportunity. That is why it is a good idea to have some sort of documentation process to record when opportunities are introduced by phone, letter or e-mail and who introduced them.

WHAT ABOUT LICENSURE AND HOSPITAL PRIVILEGING?

These subjects are addressed in Chapters Nine and Ten.

WHAT TYPE OF MALPRACTICE INSURANCE IS OFFERED?

Malpractice is discussed in Chapter Eleven.

HOW DOES PAY WORK?

As a locum tenens physician, you are paid a daily or hourly rate that varies by medical specialty. If you direct contract you will be paid by the hospital, medical group or other organization for which you work. Those who contract through agencies are paid by the agency. Locum tenens doctors are responsible for keeping track of all hours worked, including call. Periodically throughout the assignment period (usually every other week), you submit a timesheet to your contact at the site of service, which must be approved by someone at the site. For short-term assignments, the timesheet is submitted at the end of the assignment.

WHAT CAN I EXPECT TO MAKE AS A LOCUM TENENS?

Daily rates vary and are subject to negotiation. Agencies generally do not dictate rates but arrive at a rate with the physician based on the requirements of the assignment, the physicians' credentials and supply and demand conditions in the physician's specialty and in the region. Depending on your specialty, daily rates can vary from the $500 range to more than $1,500.

Physicians can earn additional income at higher rates by working extra hours. Overtime usually begins after an eight-hour shift. You also can earn extra income by carrying a pager and being on-call. Physicians who work locum tenens on a full-time basis realize incomes that are comparable to permanent physicians working in the same specialties.

WHAT ABOUT TAXES?

As independent contractors, locum tenens physicians file Form 1099 to pay their federal taxes and can take all relevant deductions (locum tenens agencies do not withhold federal taxes when paying physicians).

You may expect to pay state income taxes, however, for income earned while working in a state that does impose state income tax, regardless of your state of residency. If your permanent home is in an income tax state, expect to pay taxes on your income no matter where you earned it.

WHAT ABOUT BENEFITS?

Agencies provide malpractice insurance but not health insurance. Locum tenens physicians must either purchase health insurance or obtain coverage through a spouse's or partner's plan.

HOW DO I GET TO ASSIGNMENTS?

This depends on the location of the assignment. You may choose to fly or drive a rental car or drive a personal vehicle. These are all details that should be negotiated with the locum tenens agency before you accept an assignment.

DO I GET TO CHOOSE MY FLIGHTS?

The locum tenens agency will discuss your flight options with you to ensure you are comfortable with all travel arrangements. At times, due to budgets set by the agency's clients, there may be certain flights that cannot be offered as an option due to cost.

IF I WANT TO BOOK MY OWN FLIGHTS, CAN I BE REIMBURSED?

If you decide to handle your own travel arrangements, you may be reimbursed by providing detailed receipts regarding flight costs. It is important that you discuss travel budgets with the locum tenens agency in advance to ensure you are reimbursed. If you wish to let the agency book your flight, the agency will pay for the flight directly and then bill its client.

IF I FLY TO MY ASSIGNMENT, HOW DO I GET FROM THE AIRPORT TO MY ASSIGNMENT?

The locum tenens agency will book a rental car for local transportation or, in larger cities, will pay for modes of public transportation.

HOW WILL I KNOW WHERE THE ASSIGNMENT IS LOCATED?

The locum tenens agency will provide a map and directions to the assignment.

IF I DRIVE MY PERSONAL VEHICLE, WILL I BE REIMBURSED FOR GASOLINE?

If you decide to drive your own vehicle to the assignment you may be reimbursed for gasoline used or paid a standard IRS mileage rate. This will be something you will need to discuss with the locum tenens agency.

WHO HANDLES MY LODGING ACCOMMODATIONS?

This may vary, but in general the locum tenens agency books accommodations for the duration of the physician's assignment. At times, the agency's hospital or medical group client may book accommodations for all locum tenens physicians working at their facilities. You may also request to book your own accommodations.

IF I HANDLE MY LODGING ACCOMMODATIONS, HOW DO I GET REIMBURSED?

If you choose to handle lodging, you have two options. You may book your hotel or apartment and be responsible for payment and then submit detailed receipts to the locum tenens agency for reimbursement. Again, make sure you have discussed lodging budgets with the agency in advance. You may also request to receive a lodging per diem (a fixed, daily amount) to cover all lodging expenses. Lodging per diems should be negotiated prior to accepting the assignment.

ARE LODGING PER DIEMS TAXABLE?

Lodging per diems are considered a non-taxable expense.

IF THE STAFFING COMPANY BOOKS MY LODGING, WILL MY REQUESTS BE CONSIDERED?

Yes. When booking the assignment, share all necessary requests and preferences with the locum tenens agency, and it should do its best to accommodate you. At times, particularly in rural areas where lodging options may be limited, it may be necessary to remain flexible about lodging.

IF THE LOCUM TENENS AGENCY BOOKS MY FLIGHT, RENTAL CAR OR ACCOMMODATIONS, HOW ARE THESE PAID FOR?

If you elect to have the locum tenens agency handle these responsibilities, the company will pay for all flights, car rentals and accommodations.

CAN I BRING MY PET TO THE ASSIGNMENT?

You may request to bring your pet on assignment. Make sure to share this request with your locum tenens agency representative up front so that they may search for pet-friendly options for your flight, rental car and accommodations. However, you will be asked to pay for any additional costs incurred because of your pet. Reasonable requests are accommodated where possible, but bringing multiple pets may not be feasible.

IF I ACCEPT A LONG-TERM ASSIGNMENT, IS AN APARTMENT AN OPTION?

Yes. The locum tenens agency will research apartment options for longer assignments—usually of one month or more. Typically, hotels are used for accommodations on assignments of less than a month.

ARE MY MEALS PAID FOR ON ASSIGNMENT?

Meals are generally not paid for on assignment. However, some clients are willing to provide meals and incidental expenses (M&IE) per diem when booking an assignment directly or through a locum tenens agency.

CAN I BRING MY FAMILY TO THE ASSIGNMENT?

You may request that your family accompany you on assignment. If additional airline tickets are necessary for your family, you will be responsible for the cost of your family travel.

CAN I USE MY FREQUENT FLYER OR REWARDS PROGRAM CARDS WHILE ON ASSIGNMENT, EVEN IF I DON'T PAY THE COSTS?

Yes. If you have a frequent flyer card or hotel rewards program card, you may give this information to the locum tenens company prior to your start date and they will submit this to the vendor for you. You are able to receive the benefits of these programs, regardless of who paid for them.

WHAT HAPPENS IF I ARRIVE AT MY HOTEL AND ACCOMMODATIONS ARE NOT ACCEPTABLE?

Call the locum tenens company to discuss your concerns and possible alternatives. A full-service locum tenens agency serves as your liaison on the assignment and should be able to help address the situation if alternatives are available.

Though these are some of the typical questions that physicians ask when considering locum tenens assignments, others inevitably arise before, during and after assignments. One way to judge the efficiency and professionalism of locum tenens firms is to see how they react to your questions and needs. A full-service firm will act as your advocate and will respond to your questions quickly. Ideally, you will develop a close working relationship with your locum tenens company representative who will serve as an organizer and expediter so that you can focus on seeing patients.

6}

ORIENTATION AND THE ASSIGNMENT

"To be prepared is half the victory."
~ Miguel de Cervantes

Locum tenens physicians, like permanent doctors, are most efficient, productive and satisfied when they are seeing patients. One of the benefits of working locum tenens is that it allows doctors to focus most of their time on patient care rather than on administrative and other non-clinical issues.

This is only the case, however, if the locum tenens doctor has been properly oriented and knows who to see and what to do. There are several steps that facilities using locum tenens physicians and locum tenens physicians themselves should take to ensure locums doctors can hit the ground running and make the most of their assignments. These include:

ASSESSMENT OF NEED

Depending on the situation, putting a locum tenens doctor in place can be a time-consuming process, particularly if the physician must be credentialed at the local hospital. Hospital credentialing times vary from as little as one day to several months. When possible, it is important for hospitals, medical groups and other facilities to plan their locum tenens needs well in advance, based on knowledge of temporary physician absences due to vacations, CME, maternity leave and other factors. If the facility has a medical staff plan that includes time frames for permanent physician recruitment, it can plan when it may need locum tenens doctors to maintain services while a permanent search is ongoing.

There will be cases involving physician illness, turnover or death for which no advance planning is possible. For this reason, it is a good idea to have a positive working relationship with one or more temporary physician staffing firms that are familiar with credentialing and other processes at the facility and can turn around assignments as quickly as possible.

PRE-ASSIGNMENT PROFILE

In permanent physician recruiting, multiple hours of communication take place between physician candidates and the facilities recruiting them before the two parties meet face-to-face. The communication bar is not quite as high in locum tenens, but pre-assignment communication still is an important part of the locum tenens process.

Staffing firms can be an asset during this process by ensuring the necessary exchange of paperwork and telephone conferences, if necessary. Whether a firm is involved or not, there are steps that should be followed to ensure that the locum tenens assignment is set up efficiently.

A productive locum tenens assignment begins with a thorough profile of the practice setting. At Staff Care, a Territory Sales Consultant reviews the assignment setting in detail with the hospital department head, medical group administrator and/or the physician for whom the locum tenens doctor will be providing coverage.

It is important that *expectations be confirmed on the front end.* The locum tenens doctor should know how many hours he or she will be expected to work each day and the number of patients he or she is likely to see. The specifics of the assignment will vary by specialty. In the case of radiology, emphasis will be placed on the type of imaging equipment available and the modalities the locum tenens radiologist will be expected to read, whether x-ray, CT, MRI, mammography or a combination of the above. The locum tenens radiologist should know approximately how many studies he or she will read per day, type of PACS available, method of dictation, whether they can cover the ED remotely from their hotel room with teleradiology or whether they must be physically present and all other related details.

With surgery, it is particularly important to determine who will conduct follow-up care. Some surgeons are reluctant to follow-up on the work of locum tenens doctors if they are not familiar with the doctor or with the concept of locum tenens in general. It is important to determine prior to scheduling the temporary assignment if follow-up care is available. It also is important to know if the hospital's bylaws require the surgeon to be board certified, as is often the case today.

One of the principal uses of locum tenens surgeons is to provide on-call services required for hospitals to maintain their trauma status level. In many cases, locum tenens surgeons will provide call coverage during nights and weekends when a local neurosurgeon, obstetrician/gynecologist, gastroenterologist or other specialist is not available. In such cases, the surgeon will remain at the hotel and be on their pagers with a required response time of 30 minutes or less. Locum tenens surgeons typically will round on hospital patients and perform surgery on unassigned patients and occasionally on assigned patients.

In primary care assignments, the locum tenens physician generally will be office based and will see the usual spectrum of patients familiar to family physicians, general internists and pediatricians. The practice profile in primary care will focus more on people than on procedures or equipment. The locum tenens physician should be familiar with the types of patients he or she is likely to see and should be provided with information regarding local specialists who are available for referrals.

Regardless of the type of locum tenens doctor on assignment, Staff Care recommends a *pre-assignment phone call* be scheduled where possible. This call will include the locum tenens physician and the physician for whom he or she is providing coverage, if appropriate. If not, the call will be between the locum tenens doctor and the practice administrator, department head or other person with the best insight into the requirements of the practice setting. The call can be a key way for the two parties to become acquainted and to get a feel for what will be required on the assignment, who the players are and the standard practices and procedures at the setting.

PRESENTATION OF CV

In a properly structured temporary assignment, the locum tenens staffing agency will not begin seeking candidates until it has conducted the practice profile. At that point, it then is in a position to identify physicians with the training, availability and disposition for a particular assignment. Most staffing firms have a pool of locum tenens physicians from which to draw—independent contractors who have either been matched with assignments in the past or who have expressed an interest in working locum tenens.

In addition to these physicians, staffing firms may source additional candidates through direct mail, Web sites, journal advertisements, convention attendance and other methods. Locum tenens staffing firms work on a contingent basis. Clients do not pay agencies until the locum tenens physician is in place providing billable services. The staffing firm's goal is to be the first to provide a qualified candidate with the required availability at a reasonable price and to ensure that clients find the locum tenens experience to be a positive one. Hospitals, medical groups and other organizations generally will choose to work with one or two such companies that have proven successful over time.

It is important to ensure during the CV presentation that the staffing firm actually is matching the physician introduced initially and not another doctor. It is a practice of some staffing firms to float the CV of a particularly impressive physician before a client. The client then suspends efforts being conducted by any other locum tenens firm in the expectation that it has a qualified doctor assigned. It then develops that the first physician is not available and another doctor is introduced—a "bait and switch" tactic that can leave the facility frustrated.

The locum tenens physician's CV generally is presented by e-mail or fax to the facility administrator, the physician he or she is filling in for or other decision makers. Staff Care conducts a background check of each physician we match with temporary assignments. Before sending a doctor on assignment, written references should be obtained and shared with the client facility.

SCHEDULING

Once the facility approves the locum tenens physician, he or she is scheduled through the staffing firm. At Staff Care, we have Account Representatives who coordinate this phase of the assignment. A first step is to determine from the hospital what is needed to credential the locum tenens physician. As referenced in Chapter Eleven, credentialing usually requires verification of the physician's work experience, education, CME and several professional references. It should be clear what the locum tenens physician is being credentialed for. In radiology, for example, the level of documentation required to credential a physician for mammography is higher than for plain film. If the locum tenens doctor is a surgeon, it may be necessary to show case logs indicating RVUs for the physician during the prior 12 to 24 months and proof of board certification.

PREPARE THE STAFF

It is a mistake to allow a locum tenens physician to show up unannounced. Explain to the staff that a temporary physician has been scheduled to provide interim coverage and to maintain quality of care and patient satisfaction. Let the staff know that the physician's qualifications have been examined and are satisfactory. Also, ask that the staff treat the temporary doctor with the same courtesy and respect that they would extend to a permanent physician.

PREPARE PATIENTS

In some cases, such as radiology or anesthesiology, it will be unnecessary to conduct patient awareness efforts. However, in primary care, it may be important for physicians or the group management to inform patients that a temporary doctor will be in place. Patients should understand the locum tenens doctor's qualifications and be informed that the use of locum tenens is a common practice in medicine today and not a cause for concern. In a hospital setting, let patients know that though the physician is a qualified substitute, everything else in the hospital, from the lead techs to the department manager, is established and has not been altered.

BILLING

Physicians will generally complete the necessary insurance forms the first day that they arrive. The DEA number should be requested during the credentialing process prior to the physician's arrival and prescription authority also should be arranged. Staffing agencies typically do not provide billing services, so it is important for healthcare facilities to consult their billing departments to ensure billing systems for the locum tenens doctor are arranged with managed care entities, Medicare and other payers. It is important to consider the requirements of payers. For example, if a managed care company requires physicians to be board certified, the locum tenens physician will need to be board certified in order to ensure payment.

If the locum tenens physician is holding a place for a physician who is temporarily absent, the locum tenens physician uses the absent physician's billing number with the appropriate modifier. If the locum tenens physician is not holding the place of a physician, then he or she will need his or her own provider number for billing purposes.

When a locum tenens physician (or any physician) begins seeing patients before their Medicare/Medicaid provider number applications have been processed, there are special modifier codes that can be used for billing. Healthcare organizations should work with their billing supervisor or outside billing agency to determine how to use special codes, bill retroactively and in general ensure that locum tenens physician services are reimbursed by third-party payers.

All services provided by the locum tenens physician are billed for through the usual channels. No third-party reimbursements for services provided by locum tenens physicians are routed to the physician or to the staffing firm.

ASSIGNMENT ISSUES/CONCERNS

It may develop that one or both parties—the locum tenens physician and/or the facility—may experience concerns or issues that need to be resolved during the assignment.

Typically, these issues may include:

- Accommodation. Most locum tenens assignments are scheduled for 30 days or less and the typical mode of accommodation is a hotel. Generally, rooms with refrigerators and cooking appliances are booked so that physicians can prepare their own meals. For longer assignments, an apartment may be arranged. Though in our experience it is an infrequent occurrence, there are instances in which local accommodations are problematic, due to factors such as location, room size, room amenities or other issues. In such cases, the locum tenens physician should ask the staffing agency to arrange for alternate accommodations. In the majority of cases, this can be arranged to the physician's satisfaction.
- Clinical/quality of care issues. Clinical methodologies and quality of care standards vary by region. There are times, though these too are limited, when a locum tenens physician will not be comfortable with quality of care standards on a given assignment. The staffing agency representative may be able to mediate and resolve these issues. However, if the locum tenens physician simply is not comfortable with the standard of care being provided, he or she may elect to leave the assignment.
- Out clause. Some locum tenens physician contracts include clauses that may penalize physicians if they decide not to go to an assignment or if they leave the assignment prematurely. It does occasionally happen that physicians decide not to provide agreed upon coverage, sometimes citing inclement weather or other reasons for not arriving at the assignment. The industry standard requires physicians to give 30 days notice if they decide not to come to an assignment or if they decide to leave before the assignment has been completed. The healthcare facility typically is required by contract to give 30 days notice if it decides it does not want the physician to come after all. It also is required to give 30 days notice if it decides to ask the physician to leave before the end of the assignment.
- Acceptance. First-time locum tenens physician often are concerned about how they will be received by patients, administrators and fellow-physicians. In our experience, courtesy and professionalism generally prevail.

In Staff Care's 2009 Review of Temporary Physician Staffing Trends, we asked locum tenens physicians about how they are received by various parties while on assignment (see below).

How are you treated by administrators, physicians and patients while on assignment?

	Accepted	Tolerated	Not Accepted
Administrators	84%	14%	2%
Physicians	86%	13%	1%
Patients	96%	3%	1%

Source: Staff Care 2009 Review of Temporary Physician Staffing Trends

OFF TIME

Locum tenens physicians are expected to be on-call or on site performing services for a set number of hours stipulated in the contract. Once these hours are over, physicians are free to explore the community or otherwise do what they like. Hospitals may have codes of conduct they expect doctors to abide by and it is important for physicians to maintain a high level of professionalism.

PERMANENT POSITION

It is not unusual for locum tenens physicians to be offered a permanent job by the hospital or medical group for which they are providing coverage. If the physician accepts, the hospital or medical group generally is required by contract to provide the locum tenens agency with a placement fee.

WRAP-UP

At the end of the assignment period, the locum tenens physician is usually asked to complete all charts and provide all signatures where necessary. On some locations, the physician may be given an after-the-fact online option for doing this. The staffing agency may call the physician and its client for a post-assignment evaluation.

PAYMENT

As referenced earlier, the physician is given a form at the beginning of the assignment to track his or her hours and submit invoices to the staffing agency. Invoices and payments are typically sent bi-weekly.

Like any form of medical practice today, paperwork and "bureaucracy" are not absent in locum tenens. However, the role of the staffing agency is to reduce the hassle factor for both physicians and clients, streamlining the process and making it as efficient as possible. In addition, everything is relative. Many physicians find locum tenens to be a comparatively burden-free style of practice and embrace it for that reason.

Those who want a more detailed discussion of the mechanics of locum tenens, including a look at licensure, hospital credentialing and malpractice, may wish to read the concluding chapters of this book, which address those topics. In the next two chapters, however, we will introduce you to both some amazing country doctors and to physicians who have stories to tell about locum tenens practice.

7}

MEET THE "COUNTRY DOCTORS OF THE YEAR"

> ***"When we quit thinking primarily about ourselves and our self-preservation, we undergo a truly heroic transformation of the consciousness."***
> ~ **Joseph Campbell**

Once there was a time when physicians knew their patients intimately and when continuity of care wasn't measured in months or years but in generations. During this golden area, a patient's family doctor was equal parts psychiatrist, obstetrician/gynecologist, pediatrician, surgeon and sometimes, father confessor.

That was, of course, in the far-off "good old days" before managed care, treatment protocols, specialization and the rise of malpractice.

Or was it?

Though it may come as a surprise to lay people and even to some physicians, the classic, old-time family doctor is not a relic from the past. Marcus Welby still lives in our nation's rural communities.

There are still old-style country doctors who have cared for their patients for years and who have cared for their patients' children and even grandchildren. These doctors still round on their patients in the hospital, keep office hours, deliver babies, perform minor surgery, take care of nursing home patients and even make house calls. On occasion, they are still paid in kind—with pies, produce and other gifts.

But their numbers are dwindling. According to the National Rural Health Association, more than 20 percent of the U.S. population resides in rural areas, but fewer than 11 percent of the nation's physicians practice in the country. The demographics are not favorable. Sixteen percent of rural physicians are over 65, compared to 13 percent of all physicians. Who will replace these older doctors when they retire or die?

The answer to this question is very much in doubt. Merritt Hawkins & Associates conducts a survey every other year of medical residents in their final year of training. One of the questions they ask of young doctors "coming out" is where they would like to practice. Very few express a preference for smaller, rural communities (see below):

Based on population, in what size community would you most like to practice?

10,000 or less	3%
10,001 – 25,000	1%
25,001 – 50,000	13%
50,001 – 100,000	19%
100,001 – 250,000	23%
250,001 – 500,000	20%
500,001 – 1 million	15%
Over 1 million	6%

Source: Merritt Hawkins & Associates' 2008 Survey of Final Year Medical Residents

It is very difficult to attract physicians to rural practice these days for several reasons. First, the great majority of doctors train in large, urban teaching hospitals. They are accustomed to having a lot of technical resources at their disposal and many specialists on site for back up. Many are leery of being thrown out on their own in rural America. In addition, the hours and practice style can be more demanding, particularly because they have to be on-call more often than urban doctors. And most doctors want the same things from a community that other professionals want—movie theaters, restaurants, opera companies, professional sports and other amenities that the country sometimes can't offer.

Perhaps the biggest impediment to attracting physicians to rural areas is what is known as "trailing spouse syndrome." In the "old days" physicians were predominantly male and they were the sole breadwinners in the family. Today, many physician spouses—both male and female—also are professionals such as lawyers, accountants, computer programmers, writers, architects, etc. While there is plenty of work in smaller communities for physicians, there often is little work for their spouses. Attracting a physician to a community really means attracting his or her whole family. No work for the spouse—or inadequate amenities for the children, such as a top ranked gymnastics program or a renowned piano instructor—can be a recruitment deal killer and often is.

For this reason alone, doctors are likely to be in short supply in rural America for the foreseeable future.

Staff Care has a particular interest in and admiration for country doctors stemming from the early years of our company when many of our clients were based in rural areas. The locum tenens industry itself was started by federal grants aimed at increasing physician access in rural areas and this was Staff Care's primary focus in the early 1990s. At that time, it was mostly rural communities that needed temporary doctors to fill in while permanent physicians were being sought. Facilities in urban areas generally used locum tenens, if at all, to fill in for temporarily absent physicians.

As referenced in Chapter One, the physician market has changed considerably in recent years and physician shortages have become pervasive in many areas, urban, rural and suburban. Staff Care's clients today are as likely to be in a top 10 metropolitan area as they are to be in Mayberry, RFD. Nevertheless, we still feel committed to areas where the physician shortage always has been the most acute—rural America.

It is for this reason that Staff Care chose to highlight the accomplishments of rural practitioners and to promote rural medical practice through the *"Country Doctor of the Year℠ Award."* Every year, Staff Care receives nominations for this award, submitted by healthcare professionals or average citizens of small towns nationwide wishing to honor their country doctors. Winners of the award have been profiled nationally in media outlets that include *People* magazine, *Parade, USA Today* and "The Today Show."

These are all outstanding medical practitioners who exemplify the spirit, skill and dedication of the country doctor, and we would like to introduce them to you.

14 GREAT COUNTRY DOCTORS

In chronological order, the Country Doctors of the Year are:

John Harlan Haynes, Country Doctor of the Year, 1992

Vivian, Louisiana
Population: 4,156

Described by his patients as "a cross between Daniel Boone and Marcus Welby," Dr. Haynes has practiced in this rural community for more than 35 years, single-handedly keeping the hospital open. Renowned for his diagnostic ability, Dr. Haynes is known as a friend and a lifesaver throughout eastern Louisiana.

Claire Louise Caudill, Country Doctor of the Year, 1993

Morehead, Kentucky
Population: 8,357

Known as "The Mother of Rowan County," Dr. Caudill, now deceased, delivered more than 8,000 babies in her 50-year career and was noted for her house calls to people in the "hollers" of rural Kentucky. Dr. Caudill is a legend in her region of the state. Both a play and a book have been written about her and St. Claire Hospital in Morehead was named in her honor.

William Hill, Country Doctor of the Year, 1994

Carrolton, Alabama
Population: 1,170

"Dr. William" served as a solo physician in Carrolton for more than 50 years, carrying on a family tradition. Hill family physicians have served Carrolton continuously since before the Civil War.

Elton D. Lehman, Country Doctor of the Year, 1996 (no candidate selected in 1995)

Mount Eaton, Ohio
Population: 250

For 34 years, Dr. Lehman brought modern medicine to the Amish community of Stark County, while also serving as the town's mayor. Dr. Lehman helped design, fund and build a freestanding birthing center for Amish women as a safer alternative to home delivery. The center features a hitching post for horses and buggies and gas rather than electric lamps to help Amish patients feel more comfortable. Dr. Lehman is the author of a well-received book on country medicine called *House Calls and Hitching Posts* in which he relates stories about practicing rural medicine among the Amish. Dr. Lehman has become active in the Country Doctor of the Year Award selection process and has served on the award's selection committee helping to evaluate nominations and interview and select nominees.

Paul F. Maddox, Country Doctor of the Year, 1998 (no candidate selected in 1997)

Campton, Kentucky
Population: 525

Dr. Maddox treated more than 1.5 million patients during his 47-

year career. During much of that time he was the only physician serving an entire county, treating many patients free of charge. Dr. Maddox kept his clinic open 24 hours a day, 365 days a year for two decades—while serving as the town's mayor. He continues to practice at age 74 even after being diagnosed with cancer, scheduling patients around daily chemotherapy.

Howard Clark, Country Doctor of the Year, 1999

Morton, Mississippi
Population: 4,000

At age 73, Dr. Clark still works more than 90 hours a week, covering his clinic practice, the hospital emergency room, the nursing home and making house calls. He was largely responsible for reopening the county hospital and once covered the emergency room for 23 consecutive days—at no charge. Dr. Clark routinely treats patients regardless of their ability to pay and did not miss a local high school football game for which he was the team doctor from 1956 to 2000.

Kamlesh Gosai, Country Doctor of the Year, 2001 (no candidate selected in 2000)

Bentleyville, Pennsylvania
Population: 2,700

Prior to recruiting Dr. Gosai, Bentleyville had tried to recruit a physician without success, though they were offering a new building with rent-free office space and financial incentives. When Dr. Gosai set up shop in 1988, he declined all incentives and simply got to work. He now sees more than 300 patients a week regardless of their ability to pay and he has recruited six other doctors. Residents credit him for saving a dying town by restoring healthcare services, developing a medical laboratory with MRI and spearheading the creation of an industrial park. In his "spare time" he visits 21 nursing and personal care homes and makes hospital rounds.

James Blume, Country Doctor of the Year, 2002

Forest Hill, West Virginia
Population: 75

Diagnosed with colon cancer in 2001, Dr. Blume ignored the effects of chemotherapy and kept treating patients at his small town clinic. At times he was so weak he leaned against walls for support while working. Yet he also broke ground on an urgent care center 14 miles away and volunteered to deliver four sermons a week after a nearby church lost its pastor. Despite a malpractice crisis that drove many physicians away from West Virginia, Dr. Blume chose to sell a bit of property in order to cover insurance costs so he could continue providing care to residents of Forest Hill.

Charles Boyette, Country Doctor of the Year, 2003

Belhaven, North Carolina
Population: 1,968

When Hurricane Isabel descended on North Carolina, many people fled. Dr. Boyette gathered up medical supplies and prepared his home to serve as a temporary emergency room, treating a variety of injuries and a heart attack. This is illustrative of Dr. Boyette's commitment to Belhaven, where he rescued the local hospital from bankruptcy, launched a foundation providing financial aid to more than 100 community college students and served as major. And he still makes house calls.

Kenneth Paul Mauterer, Jr., Country Doctor of the Year, 2004

Olla, Louisiana
Population: 1,417

"Doctor Kenny Paul," as he is known to the residents of Olla, is a true homegrown hero. The community helped put Dr. Mauterer through medical school and he returned the favor by practicing in his hometown for the last 30 years, single-handedly keeping the local hospital open for much of that time.

Katrina Poe, Country Doctor of the Year, 2005

Kilmichael, Mississippi
Population: 900

Raised in the tiny community of Kilmichael, Dr. Poe returned to her hometown after her residency and now is the only physician in Kilmichael. On-call virtually 24 hours a day, Dr. Poe maintains a remarkable schedule, caring for the people of Kilmichael while also maintaining her role as a wife and mother. Young and African-American, Dr. Poe represents a new generation of country doctors.

David Nichols, Country Doctor of the Year, 2006

White Stone, Virginia
Population: 400

Dr. Nichols has been a country physician serving the small town of White Stone, Virginia, for almost 30 years. He has gained renown, however, as "Doctor Copter," since for more than 25 years he has flown out to miniscule Tangier Island in a helicopter once a week to care for its unique population. Located in the Chesapeake Bay, Tangier Island was settled in Captain John Smith's time and its population of 600 is still studied by linguists interested in Elizabethan English.

Dr. Nichols has been essential to the island's wellbeing, saving many lives and starting a drive to build a new clinic on the island. This effort received a considerable boost from the attention Dr. Nichols received through the Country Doctor of the Year Award, including a feature story in *USA Today* and a profile on national television news. Dr. Nichols and the clinic's Steering Committee have since raised $1.5 million for the clinic and construction is scheduled to begin in the summer of 2009. In addition, the clinic will be staffed by a full time physician assistant who is a resident of Tangier Island that Dr. Nichols groomed for a medical care. Dr. Nichols also served on the Selection Committee for the 2008 Country Doctor of the Year Award.

Hiram Ward, Country Doctor of the Year, 2007

Murfreesboro, Arkansas
Population: 2,000

Dr. Ward served as Murfreesboro's physician for more than 50 years. He made national news in 2007 when, at the age of 81, he came out of retirement to save the local hospital after it lost all the physicians on its staff. Dr. Ward was the only doctor providing coverage at the hospital and was on call seven days a week, 24 hours a day, accepting no salary from the hospital for these duties. Through his extraordinary and life-saving efforts, Dr. Ward has been instrumental in maintaining the hospital, which provides the foundation for both healthcare and economic viability for the community.

David H. Watson, Country Doctor of the Year, 2008

Yoakum, Texas
Population: 6,000

When Dr. Watson began practicing family medicine in 1958 in Yoakum, Texas, he charged $3 for an office visit and $5 for a house call. He also would accept payment in the form of a bushel of pecans, the haunch of a deer or an apple pie. Much has changed since then, but in many ways Dr. Watson has remained the same. He still makes house calls, still accepts payment in kind and still is the lynchpin of healthcare in his community, seeing 25 to 300 patients a day at age 78. He also rounds on hospital patients, is medical director of the nursing home and provides free care to the children at the local home for abused and neglected youth. It is no wonder that Yoakum Community Hospital has named a wing of the facility in Dr. Watson's honor.

VANISHING LEGENDS

What most of these legendary doctors have in common, in addition to their extraordinarily high commitment to their patients, is that they are 70 years old or older, already retired or deceased. Only Drs. Blume, Gosai, Mauterer and Poe are likely to provide medical care to their communities for the long term.

Who will replace these great country doctors when they are gone? The answer to that question remains very uncertain.

8}

TALES FROM THE ROAD

> ***"The road goes ever on and on, down from the door where it began."***
> ~ **J.R.R. Tolkien**

WHAT'S IT LIKE OUT THERE?

In this book we have explained some of the characteristics of locum tenens practice and reviewed various logistical and other practical matters pertaining to temporary medical practice.

To get a feel for what locum tenens practice is really like, however, you need to hear from doctors who have actually taken their medical bags on the road. Following are stories provided to us by locum tenens doctors that offer a glimpse of what it's like when your calling card reads, *"Have stethoscope, will travel."*

"Rocking the Pentagon"

~ Cherilynn Romano, Ph.D.

I have had so many adventures working locum tenens for Staff Care, I hardly know where to start. I've walked different parts of the Appalachian Trail, visited Jamestown and Williamsburg, Virginia, won a Texas Hold 'Em card tournament in Atlantic City, New Jersey, and used a big chunk of my winnings to take good friends (made on the job) to dinner at The Capitol Grill in Washington, D.C. I've enjoyed lunches with real rocket scientists from NASA when working at Fort Eustis, Virginia. I've met representatives from the NSA, CIA, FBI, etc. during a training day on the role of psychology in the intelligence community. I've even visited the International Spy Museum in Washington, D.C., but the best of all was getting the opportunity to give a presentation at the Pentagon!

There are always some problems that may take some patience or creativity to deal with, but Staff Care has always been by my side in solving issues. My mom died while I was working on the East Coast. The Staff Care logistics wizards got me a ticket for a decent price in less than 24 hours so I could get to Arizona. On my own, I would have managed to get a flight but I would have paid a huge last-minute booking price. It was just a comfort to have a team that really helped me deal with that ordeal.

At every site I have made long-lasting friendships—I'm even vacationing in Aruba with two locum tenens-made friends this December.

I have also expanded my knowledge base. Where else would I have been exposed to Navy CSI Psychological Autopsies seminars? I have biked the monuments in Washington, D.C., spent the Fourth of July at the National Mall with a vet who had never been able to go to fireworks celebrations since the Vietnam War. I have increased my understanding of what our military men and women endure in their service to all of us. I understand our politics and military better and have grown personally in knowing so many brave soldiers and Marines.

The Pentagon? THE BEST!

"Locum Tenens: A Cultural Experience"

~ Jose Carranza, M.D. (Psychiatry)

I have been doing locum tenens since 2007. I've done assignments in Santa Maria, California; Ventura, California; Brownsville, Texas; and Gouverneur, New York. Each of my assignments have been between two and three months long and have been in both outpatient and inpatient settings.

I found it interesting that most of the patients in Brownsville, Texas, only spoke Spanish and they complained that before seeing me, they had English-speaking psychiatrists who did not understand anything the patients told them and in spite of that, they were given medications. The patients there were really happy and were able to speak out all their feelings and problems in their own language with me (I am bilingual). I also met two patients who were already "labeled" as mental patients who were not really patients, but were attending that clinic because of the lack of understanding in previous meetings and evaluations. One of them was "declared mentally ill" because she wanted to sing and play music and actually she was a musician, sang with groups and did really well.

I believe that in all clinical settings, what is most important is to practice good medicine, make good diagnoses and treat the right conditions with the right medications. This is true for locum tenens as well as for any permanent jobs.

I enjoyed the weather and the warm people in Gouverneur.

Gouverneur is a very small town of about 5,000 people, but in the clinic there I saw patients from about 14 other towns that are located within the catchment area of this particular mental health center. The patients, although poor, were very intelligent and assertive. I enjoyed very intelligent conversations with several college graduates attending the clinic in Gouverneur.

Locum tenens jobs have allowed me to see new places in America. I was so impressed in Santa Maria to be able to walk on their beautiful beach in Guadalupe, California, and admire those great dunes and all their bird sanctuaries. I also enjoyed visiting on weekends the Oso Flaco Lake area, also on the coast of central California. Thanks to two locum tenens assignments in central California, I had the opportunity to eat at wonderful restaurants in Morro Bay and visit the Hearst Castle. When in Gouverneur, my wife and I visited Canada often and spent three weekends in Ottawa and Montreal, where we were able to admire their religious art.

So, in summary: Locum tenens work is the same as permanent jobs, except that you can travel and meet new people and treat a variety of patients from different parts of American cultures.

"Keep the Patients, Lose the Call"

~ James Long, M.D. (Family Practice)

Prior to locum tenens work, I practiced in a rural area for more than 40 years. When I retired I was ready to give up the call, but not contact with patients, so I started doing fill-in work for various locum tenens companies and have enjoyed doing just clinic work—especially leaving at the end of the day and not having to carry a beeper.

I have worked in a locum tenens capacity since I retired in 1995 and have worked in many interesting places and met a lot of wonderful people. Also, my wife accompanies me and enjoys becoming familiar with different areas of the Midwest. Most of my work has been short-term, but I did work for a month at Offutt Air Force Base and enjoyed working with military personnel, although it was different. It was great working with young enthusiastic people. I worked at one clinic that was right on the Mississippi close to a casino and sometimes some of the personnel would race down to the casino and play blackjack over their noon hour.

Most of my work has been in smaller communities in Nebraska and Iowa, and most of my enjoyment has been working with different people and meeting interesting patients. One of the drawbacks has been the lack of follow-up of some of the interesting cases I've seen. I think locum tenens practice has been very interesting for me and for my wife, and I think it would be a great satisfaction to anyone who is about to retire or for a doctor who has just finished training and is looking for a place to establish a practice.

"Adventures in Cowboy Country"

~ Bev Reeves-Dudley, CRNA, MA

I started doing locums since 1994. At that time, I wanted to form my own company so that I could put away a maximum amount of retirement money and the business arrangements working for local corporations were not adequate. My first assignment was down in Wichita, Kansas, for five months. I worked for a great group of doctors and CRNAs until the company was taken over and dissolved into another competing group. Interstate 35 south of Emporia, Kansas, is unbelievable prairie and the Flint Hills. There were wide-open ranges sculpted by forces of nature that had left stark, uninhabited, rolling bluffs. I saw a sign that said 'antelope restoration project.' One morning I saw a highway patrolman pulling a dead antelope off of the highway. I never saw any others. The other sign of interest was the 'prairie burning' warning. I took my bicycle with me and rode the local trails after work.

My next assignment was in Kansas City doing maternity leave coverage. My interview was the best I've ever had. My new anesthesiologist CEO was of German birth. I took German in high school and never had found any use for it until this job. The CEO had been a U.S. citizen for many years but he allowed me to practice my language in conversation with him when things weren't busy. I basically did the eye room and a smattering of everything else. That hospital became a casualty of mismanagement and the clientele had changed to more jobless without insurance over the years. I stayed there four years. It was painful to watch the place fail financially.

My next assignment was an emergency relief out in western Kansas. I took the train from Kansas City to a town one hour away. It was an all-night train ride. I then rented a car and went to my assignment past wheat fields on all sides of the road. My new anesthesiologist CEO was originally from Poland and was very sensitive, smart and easy to work with. I was glad to help out. They were stretched thin even before the emergency opening. The hospital CEO greeted me at the door to the OR. I was able to do epidurals again, which my previous locum assignments hadn't allowed. I actually got an orientation from the head CRNA and was able to hit the ground running with more ease. My fill-in time out there was sporadic but always gratifying over the years. I took the scenic route out there one time by car and found Carrie Nation's house and some geological formations of interest. I always looked for the first tumbleweed. The motels had Western names and themes—I was in cowboy country.

"Locums Work Not Hard to Swallow"

~ George Bunch, M.D. (Pediatrics)

I have worked locum tenens for one year since retiring from my private practice of 35 years in Las Vegas, New Mexico. I have mostly worked for two local solo practice pediatricians in Watsonville, California, and Capitola, California, to allow them time off. This work has ranged from two days to two weeks at a time.

The two weeks' work was for one pediatrician's trip with his wife to her homeland and for Lenten Carnival Festival in Brazil. My only work outside the Bay Area was two weeks in Carlsbad, New Mexico, for Staff Care, covering for a solo practice pediatrician on vacation to his native India.

My two weeks in Carlsbad, was 30 miles from my hometown of Artesia, New Mexico. During the visit I saw high school classmates and visited with cousins who I had not seen in 45 years. I toured the Carlsbad Caverns and Sitting Bull Falls Recreation Area, both favorite haunts of my childhood years. Each afternoon I would jog along the Pecos River Town Lake Park past my former (1950s) Boy Scout Aquatic Camp and waterfront activities from my days in Scouting, including taking my own Boy Scout Troop from Las Vegas in the mid 1980s.

In Carlsbad I saw an 8-year-old gymnast with chest pain sudden onset during running at school during recess. She was anxious but in no distress and said the pain was better and that she had no respiratory symptoms. Her exam was normal including BP, pulse, temp, but family history revealed that her grandparents had both died in their 50s from heart trouble and an uncle had heart surgery as a child and required continuing cardiac care for unknown reasons. A call to a pediatric cardiologist in Albuquerque, New Mexico, recommended that we get an ECG, but that he doubted that this was a cardiac problem. After arriving at the hospital for ECG, the child or a friend revealed that she had fallen off the monkey bars at school, so a chest x-ray was obtained. The x-ray showed a large round foreign body in mid-sternum. The child then admitted that when she fell off the monkey bars she had swallowed a quarter!!! The quarter was removed and the child did well!

During locums work I have enjoyed meeting new people and helping them through various childhood illnesses, well child care and other issues. During my work in Carlsbad it was especially interesting to meet many patients from my hometown of Artesia, many of whom had received medical care and some even were delivered by my father who was a general practitioner in Artesia for 40 years. While there I attended one of my high school's football games, where I saw several former classmates.

One drawback of locums work is not knowing the patients, their illnesses and the referral facilities and providers in the area. I would recommend locums work to anyone who enjoys new adventures, is friendly, likes to meet new people and is willing to improvise with limited or unknown resources.

"From Eight Weeks to Seven Years"

~ Amanda Weiss, M.D. (Psychiatry)

In February 2002 I accepted a locum tenens assignment for a short period—eight weeks, I think—but the two months quickly turned into six and then I was offered the permanent position at the hospital. According to the contract, Staff Care was entitled to a finder's fee, which the hospital was not prepared to produce and which I did not have. I called Staff Care and explained that after completion of all the initial assignments for which I was contracted, the contract had always been extended—and in most cases because of how pleased the hospitals were with the work I did, they decided from then on to work only with Staff Care. Hence, Staff Care had made good money from me and increased its excellent reputation as well.

I had been offered a permanent position in the past, but no place had really caught my interest like this one had. For the most part, the people I had met there were very nice, the area surrounding the hospital seemed like a safe environment conducive to raising children, with good schools, etc.

In summary, I had been looking like a hen for the right place to hatch my egg and I had found it. So for all the above reasons I requested that Staff Care consider waiving the finder's fee—and to my surprise and the hospital's, they did. I am forever grateful for such generous, selfless action. February 2009 marks the seventh year that I have been at this hospital.

9}

THE LICENSING PROCESS

> *"A license cannot be revoked because a man is red-headed, except for a calling in which red-headedness may have some rational bearing."*
> ~ **Felix Frankfurter**

While many physicians find locum tenens practice to be refreshingly free of bureaucratic hassles, there is no such thing as paperless medicine. Some level of paperwork is required, particularly when it comes to licensure, before physicians work locum tenens assignments.

It is, of course, a legal requirement for physicians practicing locum tenens in a given state to have an active medical license in that state. The exception is for physicians taking locum tenens assignments in federal government facilities, such as a Veterans Affairs (VA) Medical Center, an Indian Health System facility or a naval hospital. In such cases, physicians are able to maintain one active state medical license and practice in any of the 50 states.

If a physician does not have a license in the state where he or she would like to accept a temporary assignment, then a license must be obtained. Physicians can apply for state licenses on their own. However, some full-service locum tenens agencies will help obtain state licenses on the physician's behalf. Staff Care, for example, maintains a large in-house licensing department that helps physicians to obtain state licenses and meet hospital credentialing requirements.

This is one key for physicians who wish to *make themselves marketable* as locum tenens doctors. The more state licenses physicians hold, the more opportunities they can accept with the least amount of processing times and delays. Physicians with multiple active state licenses are in great demand and usually find it easy to maintain a full-time schedule of locum tenens assignments. Other physicians who prefer to work locum tenens in a limited geographical area maintain one or two state licenses and still may be able to schedule as many assignments as they wish to work, generally closer to home.

During the course of the last 16 years, Staff Care has developed working relationships with the various state licensing boards and usually can help expedite the process, which is characterized by regional variances in terms of filing fees, paperwork requirements and turnaround times.

A full-service locum tenens company typically will cover the entire cost of obtaining the license necessary for the specific assignment a physician has accepted.

TOUGHER STANDARDS

As was mentioned in previous chapters, locum tenens physicians were not as generally accepted decades ago as they are today. One reason that temporary doctors are more widely accepted today is that licensing and credentialing standards have become more complex and structured. These standards do not just apply to temporary physicians. Increasing public demand for protection, coupled with the growth in the number and sophistication of fraudulent practitioners over the past two decades, has resulted in stronger and more complex licensing boards and licensing statutes throughout the country. (See AMA.com for more information)

Like most locum tenens staffing firms, Staff Care provides malpractice insurance to the physicians it matches with temporary assignments. It is therefore in the interest of staffing firms to ensure locum tenens physicians are well qualified, licensed and credentialed.

The licensing/credentialing process accomplishes the following:

- Ensures that physician' 'credentials and background are verified and that they are not on record as being a threat to the public.
- Certifies a physician's ability to apply knowledge, concepts and principles and to demonstrate fundamental patient-centered skills that are important in health and disease and that constitute the basis of safe and effective patient care.
- Achieves the social benefit of protecting the consumer by maintaining minimum standards for entry into the profession.
- Complies with laws that were enacted under the police power reserved to the states by the U.S. Constitution to protect the health, safety and general welfare of their citizens. These laws give the states the ability to effectively monitor the quality of persons wishing to practice medicine in their areas.

LICENSURE BY PHYSICIAN TYPE

There are a variety of permutations in the licensing process that may vary by the physician applicant's status. Following is a breakdown of licensure considerations based on physician status:

New medical graduates

From a licensing perspective, physicians just out of training have some advantages when it comes to obtaining licensure. These include:

- Limited work history to verify. Because of their minimal track record, it is easier to verify the work history of residents than of more experienced physicians.
- The majority of new graduates do not have malpractice/background issues that must be explored.
- New graduates recently completed either the last portion of the licensing exam, i.e. USMLE or NBOME or were recently board certified, so there is no need to worry about the 10-year rule, which requires that if a physician has not passed a licensing exam or met alternative requirements (which vary by state), he or she must sit for the Special Purpose Exam (SPEX.)

International medical graduates (IMGs)

The licensure process is more involved for IMGs in part because it must be ensured that their overseas medical education is approved by the state medical licensing board in the state where the locum tenens assignment will take place. The World Health Organization (WHO) is the entity that verifies whether or not an overseas medical school is approved.

Some states allow IMGs to demonstrate that their medical education is equivalent to that of an American medical graduate. One way to do this is to go through the American Association of Collegiate Registrars and Admissions Officers (AARCO). AARCO conducts additional research to prove that the medical graduate's education was equivalent to U.S. medical education. However, not every state allows applicants to do this.

Each state requires some sort of documentation from the IMG's medical school, whether it is verifying the applicant's medical education, obtaining a certified copy of his or her medical transcripts or verifying clinical clerkships.

The time it takes to get a license can be longer for IMGs than U.S. graduates due to the fact that they have to obtain verifications from overseas.

IMGs have to obtain verification from the Educational Commission on Foreign Medical Graduates (ECFMG) that they have obtained ECFMG Certification by passing the various exams required and by fulfilling ECGMG's medical education credential requirements.

The Federation Credentials Verification Service (FCVS) was established in September 1996 to provide a basic profile in a uniform fashion for state medical boards to obtain a verified, primary source record of a physician's medical credentials. Because the verification process is relatively more complicated for IMGs, using FCVS makes particular sense for IMGs. However, some 17 states require *all* physicians to use FCVS.

By using FCVS, credentialing staff at hospitals and other institutions need only submit one verification of training or education per physician, rather than duplicating the process every time a new state license is required. The physician's record is stored permanently on site as well as off site for reproduction, review and audits. Files are maintained both electronically and by paper file.

FCVS obtains primary source verification of personal identification, pre-medical education, medical education, postgraduate training, examination history and board certification for both U.S. medical graduates and IMGs.

Locum tenens physicians

A common licensing scenario takes place when a physician practicing locum tenens wishes to obtain a license in a state where he or she currently is not licensed in order to accept an assignment in that state. There are several factors to consider in this scenario.

Most states require verification of hospital privileges that the physician held within the last five years. There are some states, however, that require verification of hospital privileges that the physician held within the last 10 years.

The higher the number of hospital privilege verifications that must be obtained, the longer it may take to obtain the license. Depending on how quickly the physician is needed, experienced locum tenens physicians who have obtained hospital privileges in many states may not be viable candidates if they can't obtain licensure in the necessary time frame. This is unfortunate since veteran locum tenens doctors understand the nuances of temporary practice and can be otherwise excellent candidates.

Another factor that can slow down the licensing process is the fact that it can be particularly difficult to verify the credentialing status of doctors who have worked at VA Medical Centers and Indian Health System facilities. The main challenge with VA facilities is that it is often difficult to get in touch with the medical staff office to process paperwork. Indian Health System locations are often in rural areas or do not have a physical mailing address but only P.O. boxes. This makes it difficult to expedite processing through the use of couriers such as FedEx, UPS or DHL since these couriers do not deliver to P.O. boxes. Verifications therefore must often be processed by the U.S. Postal Service.

Some state verification forms request that the medical director, department chairman or chief of staff at a facility where a locum tenens doctor worked complete an evaluation for the locum tenens physician's time at the facility. On occasion, this can be difficult if the assignment was only a few days and if the medical director or other doctor on site does not have a way to evaluate the locum tenens doctor's limited time spent at the facility. It is therefore important that locum tenens physicians update their CVs with each locum tenens assignment they complete, including the exact dates, addresses and contact persons at the site.

Physicians taking permanent positions and moving from one state to another

It is not uncommon for locum tenens physicians to accept permanent job offers from facilities where they have completed temporary assignments. There are various factors to consider in this scenario, including:

It may not be necessary to verify as many hospital privileges if the physician practiced in the same location for many years.

Some physicians decide to move their families before they have even begun the licensing process, not realizing that the majority of state licensure procedures are not easy, nor are they accomplished overnight. It is important for both physicians and the facilities hiring them that they do their research and understand how long the process is likely to take before the physician moves. Many physicians are put in a bind, especially when moving to states with cumbersome licensing procedures.

Military physicians

Military doctors who are transitioning to civilian practice may need to obtain a license in the state where they will be practicing, either on a locum tenens basis or in permanent positions. These doctors should keep in mind that some states such as Oregon require physicians to verify their time spent at a military base/hospital even if it was in a foreign country. The majority of states will accept an undeleted DD214 from the National Personnel Records Center.

Retired physicians who wish to "unretire" and work locum tenens or in permanent practice

If a physician is retired and wishes to begin practicing again, it can be difficult to obtain a license because most states require that physicians be in active practice within two years of applying to the state for a license. If the physician has been out of practice for longer than a two-year period, it is up to the licensing board's discretion as to what the physician will be required to do.

TYPES OF LICENSES

There are several types of licenses for which physicians may apply whether they are working locum tenens or in a permanent position. These include:

Initial license

The initial license is for physicians who have never held a license in the state where they are going to practice, either as a locum tenens or on a permanent basis. Physicians seeking an initial license must go through the entire licensing process. All of the licensing board specific verifications must arrive for a file to be deemed complete and reviewable for a license. The initial license can be obtained by exam (first state license) or by endorsement (assuming the physician holds at least one other state license).

Inactive license

If a physician has a license in a state that has not expired but he or she does not currently practice in that state, the license may be changed to "inactive" status. In order to change this status, the physician may have to verify licenses. To have a license reactivated, physicians usually are required to obtain some additional verifications (license, Federation, National Practitioner Data Bank [NPDB], work history), depending on various state requirements.

Locum tenens license

Physicians who only intend to practice on a locum tenens basis in a particular state or states often will apply for a locum tenens license. These licenses are usually easier to obtain than other types of licenses. In some cases, the license will be site-specific and date-specific. In such cases, the physician will only be licensed to practice in a certain place during a certain time.

Some states require a statement of purpose, and the locum tenens license is good for up to 90 days at a specific site. Some states require only certain verifications for a locum tenens license while other states require all the verifications.

Not every state board offers a locum tenens license. Typically, an additional fee is required for a locum tenens license, usually in the $250 to $350 range. Some states give locum tenens licenses that are not time-specific, so a locum tenens license is good for two years and all the physician has to do is call the board and let them know the assignment site has changed.

Generally, physicians must obtain a "letter of need" from the site where the locums work will be performed before the license can be issued. The letter should indicate that there is either a shortage at the site for a particular medical specialty or need for vacation coverage.

Temporary license

In some cases, physicians will use temporary licenses to work locum tenens assignments in particular states. In others, physicians relocating to a state on a permanent basis will first obtain a temporary license to begin working in the state. Usually, the requirements for obtaining a temporary license are the same as for obtaining a permanent license, though a temporary license may be acquired more quickly, allowing the physician to practice sooner.

Keep in mind that not every board offers a temporary license.

Some states require all verifications and additional requirements (e.g., the state jurisprudence exam, background checks and personal interviews) to be complete before a physician can receive the temporary license. There are some states, however, that will allow doctors to receive the license by simply submitting an application, fee and supporting documentation.

Temporary licenses are usually valid until the state's next board meeting. There often is an additional fee necessary in order to obtain a temporary license. If a physician has to obtain a Controlled Substance Registration (CSR), some states will not allow him or her to do so with a temporary license. In these states, a permanent license will be required.

REACTIVATIONS

Some locum tenens physicians may need to reactivate licenses in states where they are accepting temporary assignments. Depending on the state and how long ago the license expired, a physician may have to apply as if he or she never held a license in the state. Usually the process requires verification of licenses and additional postgraduate training, a NPDB check, an AMA profile and any new hospital affiliations.

A license may be deemed inactive if the physician has not renewed the license and if the licensing board offers a grace period during which the license can be renewed. To have a license reactivated, physicians usually are required to obtain some additional verifications (license, Federation, NPDB, work history), depending on the state.

LICENSE RENEWAL

Physicians with expired licenses will need to have their licenses renewed. Usually it is very easy to renew a license. Most states have a paper or online application and a required fee. The form usually requires physicians to submit proof of CME hours, and the number of such hours required for renewal is determined by the board.

Generally, it takes only a couple of weeks to renew a license. Most online renewal forms ask questions that only the physician can answer (usually questions regarding discipline at either a board or a hospital), so physicians usually need to obtain renewals themselves.

TRAINING LICENSES

These licenses are for physicians seeking graduate medical education training in a particular state. A training license allows the physician to train at a teaching hospital. Physicians working locum tenens will have already obtained a training license and completed the GME.

Training licenses are fairly easy to obtain. Physicians usually only have to verify their education, previous postgraduate training, if applicable, and exam scores.

Not every state requires physicians completing their postgraduate training to obtain a training license. Such licenses only last the length of the training period.

OTHER REQUIREMENTS

Locum tenens physicians may need to fulfill other requirements beyond obtaining an active license in a particular state. These requirements may include a CSR. A CSR is a registration required by any given state for anyone who manufactures, distributes or dispenses any controlled substance within that state.

States that require a CSR for physicians include:

- Alabama
- Connecticut
- Delaware
- District of Columbia
- Hawaii
- Idaho
- Illinois
- Indiana
- Iowa
- Louisiana
- Maryland
- Massachusetts
- Michigan
- Missouri
- Nevada
- New Jersey
- New Mexico
- Oklahoma
- Rhode Island
- South Carolina
- South Dakota
- Texas
- Utah

Depending on the state, a CSR can be issued by the state medical board, state pharmacy board or the state Department of Public Health. Physicians must hold a state license before they can obtain a CSR.

If working in a state that does not offer a CSR, physicians must obtain a DEA (see below) in order to issue controlled substances.

(Radiologists are not always required to have a DEA.) If working in a state that does have a CSR, physicians first must obtain the CSR before they can obtain the DEA.

CSR is usually site specific. Physicians can call the board of pharmacy to change the site address if needed.

If applying solely for the CSR, the application process can take between a few days to several weeks, depending on varying turnaround times in given states. A CSR is usually derived through the board of pharmacy. Most states require physicians to wait until their state license has been issued before they can file the CSR application. There usually is an additional fee required in order to obtain the CSR. Staff Care covers these fees for physicians it matches to temporary assignments.

DRUG ENFORCEMENT AGENCY (DEA)

The DEA is a federal license and is not derived from the state where a locum tenens physician may be taking an assignment. A DEA authorizes a physician to prescribe medicine within the U.S. All M.D.s and D.O.s must hold a DEA in order to prescribe.

In the states that have their own state CSR, the provider is required to have the medical license as well as the state CSR before applying for a DEA in that state.

Obtaining a DEA can be done online on the DEA Web site (http://www.deadiversion.usdoj.gov/) or by sending in a paper application.

CSRs can be obtained online in some states, as well as by paper. Fees vary from state to state.

If a state requires a CSR and a DEA, the order in which they are obtained is: State license; CSR; DEA.

Some providers such as CRNAs are not required to obtain a DEA, but must obtain a CSR. Some states do not require a CSR or a DEA.

The fee to obtain a DEA is $551. Staff Care pays this fee on behalf of physicians we match if it is necessary for a particular locum tenens assignment. Physicians working in a state that offers a CSR and who receive a CSR do not necessarily have to obtain the DEA right away. However, physicians who work in a state that does not offer a CSR, will have to obtain a DEA.

Physicians can hold more than one DEA—especially if they need one that is state specific. In Idaho, for example, physicians need a DEA with an Idaho address in order to obtain a permanent CSR. Physicians working in another state will need their DEA in that state as well.

DEA offices are organized by geographic region. Some regions can process a DEA application in a few days, while others take a few weeks. Locum tenens physicians don't have to change the address of their DEA unless they will be at the facility where they are working locum tenens longer than 59 days. However, some sites require that physicians change the address of the DEA to the address of the facility where they will be on assignment before they can be credentialed.

LEGAL IMPLICATIONS

There are various legal implications relevant to the licensing process, including:

Licensing applications

It is important to ensure the malpractice and background information for doctors' applications are complete, accurate and supported by required documentation

If a physician provides a "yes" answer to a question that may involve legal implications (such as, "Yes, I have been named in a malpractice suit"), he or she should make sure that the supporting documents are sent with the initial application that is submitted to the board. Supporting documents may include the deposition in the case and the settlement/judgment.

Background checks

Hospitals, medical groups and other organizations using locum tenens physicians typically run background checks on these physicians, as do full-service locum tenens staffing agencies. A few things to consider:

- State licensing issues are reported to the NPDB.
- Criminal background checks are obtained by the state board conducting the check through fingerprint cards or by the physician's personal information (Social Security number/date of birth). The majority of medical and nursing boards are now requiring fingerprint cards.
- Fingerprint checks may take up to eight weeks to process. It is important for physicians to make the state board aware of anything that may come up before the results come in.

Revoked or suspended licenses

Obviously, there are implications for locum tenens doctors and permanent physicians when their licenses are revoked or suspended. Once a physician's license is revoked or suspended it is reported to the NPDB.

A physician must answer "yes" on all future licensing/credentialing applications when asked if his or her license has ever been revoked or suspended, which will definitely cause delays in both processes.

To obtain state licensure, physicians with revoked or suspended licenses will have to send files to a board meeting, and physicians may be required to complete personal interviews. Physicians are unable to practice medicine on a locum tenens or permanent basis during times when an investigation is being completed. Some investigations can be quite lengthy depending on the severity of the problem. If a physician holds licenses in multiple states, all of those licenses will be suspended and/or revoked until the investigation has been completed.

Licenses can be restored. Depending on the severity of the issue at hand, however, the board may elect not to restore the license. If a license is suspended, depending on the nature of the case, some boards will ask physicians to seek counseling by someone who is approved though the board. Texas, for example, requires physicians to attend courses pertaining to the cause of suspension, such as a medical record keeping course that has been approved by either the AMA or the state board.

Undisclosed malpractice issues

It may happen that during the licensing process, issues will arise that pertain to malpractice the physician did not disclose. In such cases:

- Time will be added to the licensure process.
- Most files will either be reviewed by the Executive Director or the physician will be required to attend the next Board Meeting before a permanent license can been issued.
- Undisclosed malpractice will disqualify physicians for temporary licensure if the state offers a temporary license.

If physicians do not disclose all relevant malpractice information, they will have to make addendums to their applications, and write personal statements as to what happened and why they did not disclose the information. These forms usually have to be notarized before they are sent to the board. State boards review information as though physicians are trying to deceive them, so the best thing to do is be completely forthcoming.

Most boards either request an NPDB, Board Action Report from the Federation of State Medical Boards (FSMB) or conduct a background check, so the information will come up during the process.

Depending on the severity of the issue, the board can deny physicians licensure, a fact physicians will have to report on all future licensing/credentialing applications. This will add to processing times because files will have to be reviewed.

Physicians named in malpractice suits should keep copies of court documents because medical boards want to examine the deposition and settlement. Not having them can delay issuance of the license.

HOW LONG WILL IT TAKE?

Whether seeking a license for locum tenens work or for a permanent position, physicians, hospitals, medical groups and other facilities must consider how long the process takes. Here are a few points to consider:

- Most state licensing boards meet on a monthly basis. Some boards meet every two months. This means that if the state requires the application to be approved at the board meetings the license may or may not be issued on that date.
- Not all licenses that are reviewed at a board meeting are guaranteed to be approved or decided upon at the board meeting. It is the state board member's final decision whether or not the license will be issued at the meeting.
- The applicant's file must be complete prior to the board meeting date. Most state boards require the physician's application to be complete at least two weeks before the board meeting or it will not be considered until the next board meeting.

There are a variety of regional factors that may affect the process. For example, if a doctor has a pending malpractice suit and is applying for licensure in New Jersey, the application will go through malpractice review. This normally takes an additional six to eight weeks in this state. The malpractice review committee will determine if the application will require a board meeting.

ONE SIZE DOES NOT FIT ALL

Each state is different when it comes to licensing time frames and processes. Each state's time frames and requirements are listed on their application forms.

During peak licensing season (e.g., when physicians usually complete their residencies in May through September), board processing times often are delayed because of the increased number of applications. In the past, these delays have added up to six weeks to processing times.

There are some state boards that won't even touch an application until 30, 60 or 90 days have elapsed from the time they were received. During this time, these boards will not provide any updates on the files.

VERIFICATION REQUIREMENTS

The licensing process entails the verification of certain requirements that are necessary in order for physicians to obtain state medical licenses.

Following is a list of verifications that are required by most states. These verifications have to be "prime source generated," meaning that they cannot be faxed from the physicians, state medical board or facility. Instead, they must go straight from the facility completing the verification to the state licensing board by regular mail or courier. However, some state boards (Virginia, for example) will accept faxed verifications for hospital privileges.

License verification from another state

Obtaining verification of licensure in another state generally requires a fee ranging up to $50 and takes anywhere from one day to four weeks, depending on the state. Verification can be requested by mail. If the state board is in a "Veridoc State," physicians can request state license verification through the online Veridoc System: http://www.veridoc.org.

Initial exam score verification

A fee usually is required to obtain an initial exam score verification. Exams for which verifications may be necessary include the Examination & Board Action History Report (EBAHR) (https://secure.fsmb.org/trol/), which includes: the Federation Licensing Examination (FLEX), the Special Purpose Examination (SPEX) or the United States Medical Licensing Examination (USMLE); the National Board of Medical Examiner (http://www.nbme.org/); and the National Board of Osteopathic Medical Examiners (NBOME) (http://www.nbome.org).

Physicians also may have taken a state-constructed exam.

NPDB and Healthcare Integrity and Protection Data Bank (HIPDB) (https://icd.npdb-hipdb.hrsa.gov/RulesOfBehaviorSQ.jsp)

This background check document is available for a $16 fee and takes about two to three weeks to process. It can be ordered by physicians, medical facilities, locum tenens agencies, state medical boards and others.

Medical education transcripts

Some medical schools provide transcripts for free while others charge a fee. The process takes anywhere from two days to four weeks. During graduation season, medical schools are very busy and it could take an extra two weeks to get the transcripts to the board.

Verification of medical education

This verification can be submitted at the same time as the medical school transcript request. Depending on the medical school, both verification requests are sent to the registrar's office, though sometimes two separate requests must be sent. In such cases, one request goes to the registrar's office for the transcripts and one to the medical school for the medical education verification. Verification of medical education usually takes about five to 10 business days, depending on the school. If the doctor is an IMG, this process could take months since it can be very hard to obtain records from overseas. Time differences and language barriers can make it particularly hard to obtain these documents.

Verification of postgraduate education

This verification usually can be obtained for free, though some schools require a fee. The process can take anywhere from one day to four weeks during peak season (May through August).

Verification of educational scores (http://www.ecfmg.org/)

This requirement is for IMGs only. There is a $25 filing fee and the ECFMG usually takes about four weeks to turn this around.

Verification of employment/hospital affiliation

This is usually free and takes anywhere from a day to four weeks to process. Hospital affiliations are one of the hardest verifications to obtain. Sometimes the verifying hospital is not cooperative and occasionally the hospital will outright refuse to participate. Some verifications have taken up to three months to be returned. Some state boards only require affiliations for the past five years while others want verification of the physician's entire work history since he or she graduated from medical school. This can become one of the tedious aspects of working locum tenens. An agency like Staff Care can help alleviate this burden.

Verification of malpractice reports/insurance

In addition to the NPDB/HIPDB reports, some states require that physicians obtain verification from each malpractice carrier with which the doctor has worked. This process can take three weeks to a few months.

Verification of board certification (http://www.abms.org/)

Some boards require verification the doctor's board specialty. This can take two to four weeks depending on the specialty. The American Board of Medical Specialties (ABMS) has several member boards. To verify board specialties costs anywhere from nothing to $100. It usually takes member boards about three weeks, not counting mail time, to process verification of board certification.

Sample member boards of the ABMS include:

- The American Board of Allergy and Immunology. http://www.abai.org
- The American Board of Anesthesiology. http://www.theaba.org
- The American Board of Colon and Rectal Surgery. http://www.abcrs.org
- The American Board of Dermatology. http://www.abderm.org
- The American Board of Emergency Medicine. http://www.abem.org
- The American Board of Family Medicine. http://www.theabfm.org
- The American Board of Internal Medicine. http://www.abim.org
- The American Board of Medical Genetics. http://www.abmg.org
- The American Board of Obstetrics and Gynecology. http://www.abog.org
- The American Board of Orthopaedic Surgery. http://www.abos.org
- The American Board of Nuclear Medicine. http://www.abnm.org

- The American Board of Pathology. http://www.abpath.org
- The American Board of Physical Medicine and Rehabilitation. http://www.abpmr.org
- The American Board of Ophthalmology. http://www.abop.org
- The American Board of Preventive Medicine. http://www.theabpm.org
- The American Board of Otolaryngology. http://www.aboto.org
- The American Board of Radiology. http://www.theabr.org
- The American Board of Pediatrics. http://www.abp.org
- The American Board of Thoracic Surgery. http://www.abts.org
- The American Board of Plastic Surgery. http://www.abplsurg.org
- The American Board of Psychiatry and Neurology. http://www.abpn.com
- The American Board of Surgery. http://www.absurgery.org
- The American Board of Urology. http://www.abu.org

Disciplinary inquiry by the BSMB (http://www.fsmb.org)

This is a free verification that takes about five business days to complete.

AMA /AOA Profile

For AOA -- https://profiles.ama-assn.org/amaprofiles/ and AMA -- https://www.doprofiles.org/. The AMA profile costs $33. The AOA profile is free for doctors who are members. For non-members, the fee is $20.. This verification takes about two weeks to be returned to the board.

THE IMPORTANCE OF RENEWAL

Physicians who maintain current state licensure will be able to work locum tenens assignments much more efficiently than physicians who have to reinstate/reactivate their licenses. In order to keep licenses active, physicians should renew licenses before their expiration date. Check to see how this date varies from state to state.

Some expiration dates are on a two-year cycle, while in some states licenses expire on the physicians' birthdays. Most renewal fees are less than the initial licensure application fees. To renew a license, most state boards require physicians to provide them with a set number of

CME hours, the number of which is determined by the state board. Usually, the requirement is 100 CME hours completed within the prior two years. Usually boards require that a certain number of hours be Category 1 hours and the remaining hours can be Category 2.

CONCLUSION

As we have indicated above, the licensure process is affected by a variety of factors and can in some cases be completed quickly and with minimal hassle. In other instances, obtaining a license may be more time and resource intensive. In either case, a full-service locum tenens agency can assist in a number of ways to streamline the process and make it as efficient as possible.

Once the physician obtains a license in the state where the temporary assignment is located, the process of hospital privileging can be completed, a subject addressed in the following chapter.

10}

HOSPITAL PRIVILEGING

> *"What men prize most is a privilege, even if it be that of chief mourner at a funeral."*
> ~ **JAMES RUSSELL LOWELL**

In order to meet standards set by the Joint Commission, hospitals must confirm that physicians providing care within their facilities have the necessary credentials. Some of the credentials necessary for physicians to obtain the privilege of working at a hospital are the same ones needed to obtain licensure. For that reason, the licensure and privileging processes can be undertaken simultaneously. A physician must obtain a license, however, before the privileging process can be completed.

Full-service locum tenens agencies such as Staff Care assist with the licensing process and with the privileging process by helping to ensure that necessary documents are obtained and reviewed in a timely manner. There are a variety of documents and certifications that Staff Care's privileging department helps our clients obtain. These include:

PRIME SOURCE VERIFICATION

Staff Care's privileging department assists the medical staff office at the hospital in obtaining all types of verifications of a physician's background and credentials. Privileging coordinators send out verification requests for the physician's hospital affiliations, references and employment history at the request of the facility. Most of these verifications are sent out by fax.

BACKGROUND CHECKS

Staff Care's privileging department has the authority to run background checks on the physicians we match with various assignments per site request.

DRUG SCREENS

The privileging department can set up a drug screen test for physicians through our vendor at authorized locations throughout the country.

IMMUNIZATIONS

Physician immunization records are often part of the privileging process. Staff Care verifies that the physician is up to date on immunizations and submits results of titers if requested by the facility.

PHYSICALS

Some facilities require that the physician provide proof of a recent physical, usually within the past year. Staff Care's privileging department works with the physician to obtain this information.

NPDB REPORT

This query verifies any derogatory information on the physician. Staff Care is currently not authorized to run these types of reports but helps in requesting a self-query on behalf of the physician.

LIFE SUPPORT CERTIFICATIONS

Staff Care's privileging department will assist in verifying the physician is current in all required life support certifications (BLS, ACLS, ATLC, PALS) and send copies of the certification cards to the facility. If the physician is not up to date on these certifications, the privileging department can provide direction that will aid the physician in locating certification courses.

ONLINE COURSES

Usually these are state specific, for example, the New York State Infection Control Certification Course and Child Abuse Course. Staff Care's privileging department provides any needed information to the physician to complete these required courses.

STATE STANDARDIZED APPLICATIONS

In addition to the hospital's privileging application, a state standardized application may be required, which is a longer and more detailed application. Staff Care assists the physician in completing this application.

INTERVIEWS

Some facilities require an interview with the physician before privileges are granted. Staff Care assists in setting up the interview.

READINGS/PROCEDURAL LOGS

Depending on a physician's specialty, a facility may require additional documentation of the number of readings/procedures a physician has performed. Staff Care assists in obtaining copies of these logs from previously worked affiliations.

REPORTS

Staff Care's privileging department has the authority to run AMA or AOA profiles at the facility's request. The coordinator is also able to verify certification through the ECFMG for all IMGs.

AMERICAN BOARD CERTIFICATION

Staff Care is able to verify current American Board status through the American Board's verification system—Certifacts.

In cases where locum tenens physicians are contracting directly with hospitals or where a locum tenens agency that is not full service is involved, the hospital will need to obtain this documentation on its own. Staff Care conducts an internal process of screening physicians in which we collect much of the information needed to obtain hospital privileges, which is one reason we are able to help expedite the privileging process.

Once necessary information on the physician's background has been gathered, the hospital's privileging committee reviews the information and decides whether or not to grant the physician privileges at the hospital. There are some situations in which the locum tenens physician may be needed urgently and emergency privileges may be granted. Emergency privileges may require less thorough documentation that non-emergency privileges.

It also should be considered that some states have a standardized privileging/credentialing process that hospitals must follow. A list of these states with links to privileging/credentialing requirements and information follows:

- **Louisiana Standardized Credentialing Application** - www.ldi.state.la.us/Documents/Health/Quality_Assurance/PhysicianCredentialingForm.pdf
- **Texas Standardized Credentialing Application** - www.tsjh.org/physician-info/Credential_application.pdf
- **State of West Virginia Standardized Credentialing Form** - https://www.fghi.com/PtPortal/portals/0/Content/Careers/

WVCREDENTIALINGAPPLICATION.pdf

- **South Carolina Credentialing Application** - *http://www.i-ahc.net/custom/initial_application_southcarolina.html*
- **Integrated Massachusetts Application for Initial Credentialing/Appointment** - http://www.massmed.org/AM/Template.cfm?Section=Home&TEMPLATE=/CM/HTMLDisplay.cfm&CONTENTID=3220
- **Pennsylvania Standard Application** - https://www.keystonemercy.com/pdf/provider/provcom/credential/standard_app.pdf
- **Georgia Uniform Healthcare Practitioner Credentialing Application Form** - www.emoryhealthcare.org/departments/credentialing/pdfs/unfmap1.pdf
- **Georgia Uniform Healthcare Practitioner Credentialing Application Form for Reappointments** - www.georgiacredentialing.org/Recre.pdf
- **Maryland standard Credentialing Application** - www.phcs.com/pdf/credentialing/Maryland%20Credentialing%20Form.pdf
- **Minnesota Uniform Credentialing Application** - www.erstaff.com/collateral/FullApplication.doc
- **Oklahoma Uniform Credentialing Application** - http://www.ok.gov/health/Protective_Health/Health_Resources_Development_Service/Uniform_Credentialing_Application.html
- **CAQH (Council for Affordable Quality Healthcare)** - http://www.caqh.org/credapp/

Licensure and privileging are standard requirements for all physicians, whether they work on a locum tenens basis or in permanent practices. The same may be said of malpractice insurance, which is discussed in Chapter Eleven.

11}

COVERING YOUR TAIL

> ***"May you have a lawsuit in which you know you are right."***
>
> ~ **OLD CHINESE CURSE**

Malpractice insurance is a concern today for all physicians, whether they are in permanent practice or working locum tenens. One advantage of working locum tenens alluded to earlier is that staffing agencies usually pay for malpractice insurance on behalf of the physicians they match with temporary opportunities.

Physicians considering working locum tenens should be sure they are clear on some basic concepts regarding malpractice insurance, as should hospitals, medical groups and other users of locum tenens doctors. Following are terms and concepts to consider:

LIMITS OF LIABILITY

How much coverage do insurance carriers offer? The standard in locum tenens today is $1 million per incident and $3 million aggregate for the term of the policy, which generally is for one year. Most clients of staffing agencies and a few state medical boards request that locum tenens agencies provide this $1 million per incident/$3 million aggregate standard. Locum tenens physicians and staffing agency clients should be sure to inquire about limits of liability before working with an agency.

FINANCIAL STRENGTH/RATING OF THE CARRIER

Locum tenens physicians and those who use them should inquire into the financial strength and rating of the staffing agency's insurance carrier. Insurance carrier ratings are determined by AM Best and can be researched at www.ambest.com or on the Web site of the carrier. These ratings can be tied to the economy and general investment trends. At the time this book was written, many insurance companies had encountered financial challenges and their ratings had fluctuated.

OCCURRENCE AND CLAIMS MADE

The two main types of malpractice insurance are occurrence and claims made. Occurrence insurance covers the locum tenens physician regardless of when the claim is reported. With claims made coverage, the incident must occur and be reported while the policy is in force (again, this is typically for a one-year term).

PRIOR ACTS OR TAIL COVERAGE

Locum tenens physicians on claims made policies should make sure that the staffing agency provides prior acts or tail coverage so that the physician is protected after the policy period is over. It is important to evaluate the financial strength, longevity and track record of the staffing agency to ensure it has the wherewithal to purchase prior acts or tail coverage. If the staffing agency goes out of business, then coverage may no longer be in effect, unless the staffing company purchases unlimited tail coverage. However, if the staffing agency's insurance carrier goes out of business, the agency may seek prior acts or tail coverage elsewhere. Hospitals' and other organizations' malpractice insurance generally only covers their own employees and their acts, but not locum tenens physicians.

Facilities and practices working with locum tenens agencies also are well served to evaluate the financial strength and market position of the agencies with which they work. If neither the locum tenens physician nor the staffing agency has malpractice insurance, liability will typically fall on the hospital or medical group.

IN-STATE COVERAGE

Locum tenens physicians should be sure that the insurance carrier provides coverage in the state where the assignment is located.

PHYSICIAN ADVOCATES

If a claim is filed, the staffing agency should act as a liaison between the insurance carrier and the locum tenens physician, facilitating communication and acting as the physician's advocate.

THE FEDERAL TORT CLAIMS ACT (FTCA)

The FTCA provides a limited waiver of the federal government's sovereign immunity when its employees are negligent within the scope of their employment and generally applies to physicians working in military or Indian Health System facilities.

Link to a Clinical Handbook regarding the Federal Tort Claims Act:
- ftp://ftp.hrsa.gov/bphc/pdf/quality/2002clinicianhandbook.pdf

OTHER TYPES OF INSURANCE

Locum tenens physicians may wish to consider two other types of insurance in addition to malpractice insurance:

General liability insurance coverage

This is insurance covering the legal liability for claims of bodily injury and property damage arising out of business operations that would not be covered by the malpractice insurance policy. Examples include libel, slander and physical damage to hospital or hotel.

Workers' compensation

Since locum tenens physicians are independent contractors, they are not entitled to workers' compensation coverage from the staffing company or from the facility where they are working.

The number of claims made against locum tenens physicians is relatively low today. As in permanent practice, surgeons and radiologists are generally at higher risk for malpractice than are primary care doctors. The keys are to evaluate the insurance policies and strengths of the staffing agency and its insurance carrier and to conduct a thorough screening and orientation on the front end of the assignment so that the locum tenens physician knows what is expected, who he or she is working with and what local standards of care are.

Malpractice is an "x factor" in medical practice today for both permanent physicians and locum tenens doctors. Locum tenens physicians and the facilities that use them should take all the necessary steps to reduce risk to a minimum.

Addendum}

STAFF CARE'S 2009 REVIEW OF TEMPORARY PHYSICIAN STAFFING TRENDS

The following is a survey of healthcare facilities examining their use of locum tenens physicians and a survey of locum tenens physicians examining their locum tenens practice experiences.

Staff Care®
An AMN Healthcare Company

2009 Survey of Temporary Physician Staffing Trends

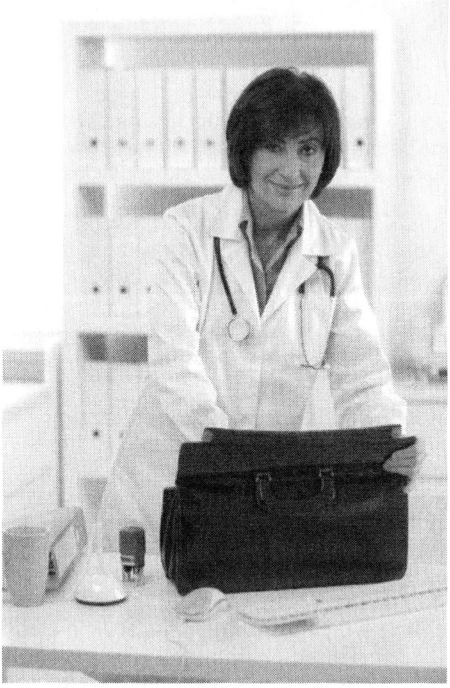

5001 Statesman Drive
Irving, Texas 75063
(800) 685-2272
www.staffcare.com

Staff Care®
An AMN Healthcare Company

Member of the National Association of Locum Tenens Organizations NALTO

Summary Report
2009 Survey of Temporary Physician Staffing Trends

Overview

Staff Care is a national healthcare staffing firm specializing in matching temporary (i.e., *locum tenens)* physicians, certified registered nurse anesthetists (CRNAs) and various allied healthcare professionals with hospitals, medical groups, government facilities and other healthcare organizations. Established in 1992, Staff Care is an AMN Healthcare company. AMN Healthcare is the largest healthcare staffing organization in the United States.

This report marks Staff Care's seventh Survey of Temporary Physician Staffing Trends. The purpose of the Survey is to track trends in the locum tenens physician staffing market and to provide benchmark data that may be useful to physicians, healthcare executives, academics, journalists and others who monitor developments in the healthcare staffing industry.

Methodology

Staff Care's 2009 Survey of Temporary Physician Staffing Trends is based on surveys sent by E-mail to healthcare executives and locum tenens physicians nationwide. The survey also includes an examination of the temporary physician staffing assignments Staff Care conducted in calendar year 2008. Data from past Staff Care surveys are included where applicable.

Part I of the survey examines why healthcare facilities, including acute care hospitals, medical groups and state-supported facilities such as behavioral health centers, use locum tenens physicians and how they evaluate the quality and services provided by locum tenens doctors.

Part II of the survey examines why physicians choose to work on a locum tenens basis, how they select temporary practice opportunities, how long they intend to work on a temporary basis, how they are perceived by colleagues, and related matters.

Part III of the survey indicates the type of locum tenens staffing assignments Staff Care conducted in calendar year 2008. The breakdown of temporary physician "days requested" by specialty is offered as an indicator of current physician supply and demand trends in locum tenens. Part III also includes the number of "temporary physician days" Staff Care filled in 2008.

The Parts I and II of the survey were conducted over the four month period from April, 2009 to July, 2009. Respondents were self-selected and included both Staff Care clients and non-clients, as well as physicians who have been matched to temporary assignments by Staff Care and those who have not.

PART I

Survey of Locum Tenens Physician Users, Including Hospital, Medical Group, and Government Health Facility Managers

Number of Surveys Completed = 216

Key Findings:

Physicians have worked as locum tenens – substituting for colleagues who are absent from their practices – for many years. However, it is only in the last several decades that the use of locum tenens doctors has become widespread at hospitals, medical groups and other healthcare facilities. In the 1970s, government grants were allotted to make temporary physicians available in medically underserved rural areas, accelerating the use of locum tenens doctors.

How prevalent are locum tenens physicians in the healthcare market today? Why do healthcare facilities use temporary doctors and how do they evaluate the quality of care provided by these physicians? Part I of Staff Care's 2009 Survey of Temporary Physician Staffing Trends, completed by healthcare facility managers who use locum tenens physicians, examines these and related questions.

Key findings include:

***The use of locum tenens physicians is commonplace**. 72 percent of healthcare facilities managers surveyed indicated their facilities had used locum tenens physicians to supplement existing staff during the last 12 months.

***Facilities appear to be using more locum tenens physicians per month.** 43 percent of those surveyed said their facilities use four or more locum tenens physicians in a typical month, compared to only nine percent in 2007 and eight percent in 2005.

***More facilities are using locum tenens physicians to test market new services.** 25 percent of those surveyed said they use locum tenens physicians to test market new medical service lines, compared to only three percent in 2007 and four percent in 2005.

***The skill level of locum tenens physicians is favorably perceived.** 66 percent of those surveyed rated the skill level of locum tenens physicians as excellent or good; only 1 percent rated skill level as unsatisfactory.

***Fewer facilities are currently seeking locum tenens physicians.** *40* percent of those surveyed are currently seeking locum tenens physicians, compared to 54 percent in 2007 and 53 percent in 2005.

***Locum tenens physicians are generally accepted in the work place.** Over 50 percent of those surveyed indicated locum tenens physicians are accepted by patients, colleagues and facility administrators.

***Locum tenens physicians are generally rated as "worth the cost."** *79* percent of those surveyed indicated the value locum tenens physicians bring to their facilities is worth the cost.

An analysis of these and other findings of Part I of the survey follows survey results below.

Part I: Questions Asked and Responses Received

1. Have you used temporary (locum tenens) physicians to supplement your existing staff any time during the last 12 months?

	2009	2007	2005
Yes	**72%**	77%	79%
No	**28%**	23%	21%

2. Are you currently looking for locum tenens physicians to supplement your existing staff?

	2009	2007	2005	2004	2003
Yes	**40%**	54%	53%	51%	53%
No	**60%**	46%	47%	49%	47%

3. How difficult is it to find locum tenens coverage today compared to 12 months ago?

	2009	2007	2005	2004	2003
More difficult	**30%**	23%	20%	23%	18%
Less difficult	**14%**	16%	17%	18%	16%
The same	**56%**	61%	63%	59%	66%

4. In a typical month, how many locum tenens physicians do you use?

	2009	2007	2005
None	**37%**	38%	36%
1 - 3	**20%**	53%	56%
4 - 6	**37%**	7%	6%
7 or more	**6%**	2%	2%

5. Why do you or would you typically use a locum tenens physician?

	2009	2007	2005	2004
Fill in until a permanent doctor is found	**34%**	65%	72%	36%
Fill in for staff who have left	**22%**	61%	71%	68%
Vacation/continuing medical education	**37%**	50%	50%	54%
Meet rising patient demand	**3%**	16%	16%	13%
Fill in during peak usage times	**11%**	15%	31%	n/a
Test market a new service	**25%**	3%	4%	2%

6. What are the benefits/drawbacks of using locum tenens physicians?

Benefits	2009	2007	2005	2004
Allows continual treatment of patients	**36%**	80%	70%	76%
Prevent revenue loss	**21%**	53%	43%	44%
Prevents existing staff burnout	**16%**	34%	39%	27%
Immediate availability	**20%**	34%	54%	44%
Cost	**35%**	6%	4%	4%
Other	**6%**	6%	4%	5%

Drawbacks	2009	2007	2005	2004
Cost	**58%**	87%	81%	82%
Familiarity with department/practice	**31%**	50%	52%	45%
Learning equipment/procedures	**19%**	26%	22%	22%
Other	**15%**	18%	28%	12%

7. What is your perception of the general skill level of locum tenens physicians?

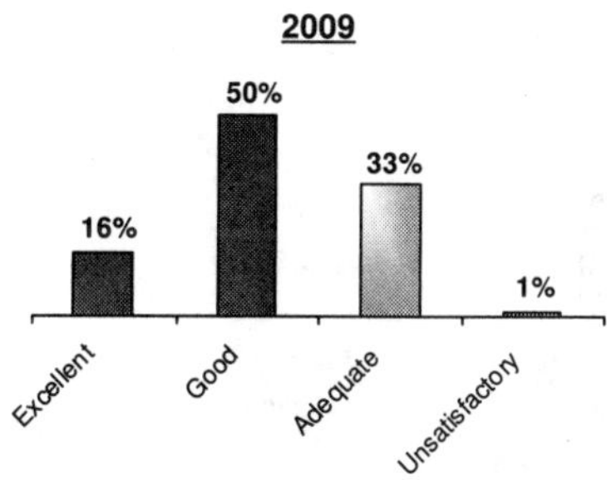

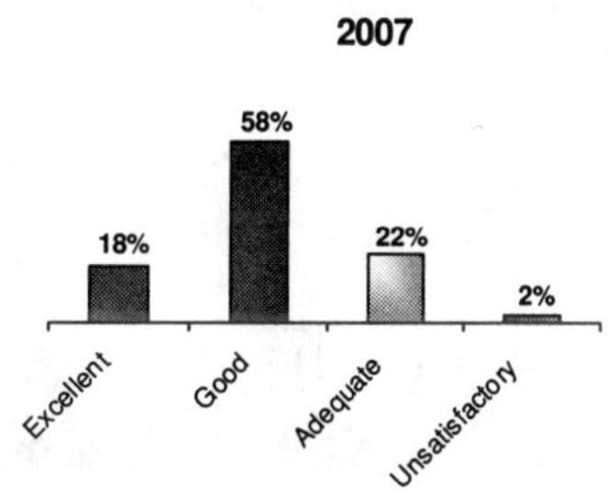

8. At your facility, how are locum tenens providers viewed by:

	2009	2007	2005
COLLEAGUES			
Accepted by	**54%**	67%	74%
Not accepted	**1%**	2%	>1%
Tolerated	**28%**	21%	16%
Unsure	**16%**	10%	11%
ADMINISTRATION			
Accepted	**57%**	68%	77%
Not accepted	**2%**	3%	>1%
Tolerated	**25%**	19%	15%
Unsure	**16%**	10%	8%
PATIENTS			
Accepted	**56%**	63%	65%
Not accepted	**0%**	1%	1%
Tolerated	**13%**	14%	17%
Unsure	**31%**	22%	17%

9. Please rate locum tenens physicians compared to your permanent medical staff in the following areas:

Patients treated per day

	2009	2007	2005	2004
More	**4%**	2%	2%	5%
Fewer	**40%**	35%	34%	26%
Same	**56%**	63%	64%	69%

10. Please rate locum tenens physicians compared to your permanent medical staff in the following areas:

Gross charges generated per day

	2009	2007	2005	2004
More	**5%**	5%	2%	3%
Fewer	**42%**	33%	37%	27%
Same	**53%**	62%	61%	70%

11. When conducting your search for locum tenens physicians, with how many search firms/ staffing agencies do you generally work?

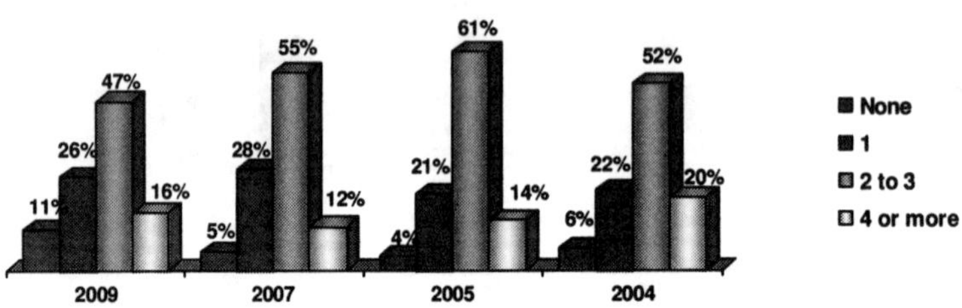

12. What are the most important factors in selecting a temporary staffing firm?

	2009*	2007*	2005*	2004
Availability of candidates/ promptness	**65%**	73%	70%	32%
Quality of physicians provided	**76%**	68%	69%	37%
Customer service	**49%**	50%	39%	7%
Cost	**52%**	49%	48%	19%
Contract flexibility	**31%**	35%	21%	2%
Malpractice insurance	**20%**	24%	16%	1%
Other	**1%**	6%	3%	3%

**Multiple responses possible in 2009, 2007, 2005*

13. How would you rate the value of locum tenens physicians to your facility?

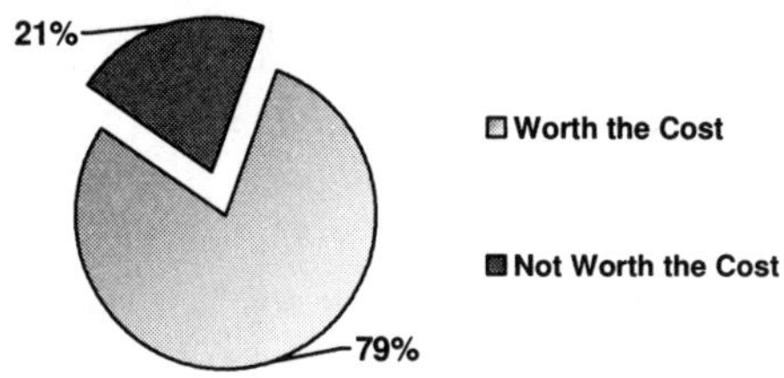

Analysis:

Part I of Staff Care's 2009 Survey of Temporary Physician Staffing Trends provides insight into how often healthcare organizations use temporary (*locum tenens)* physicians, why they use these physicians, the benefits locum tenens physicians provide, and the perceived skill levels of locum tenens physicians.

Who is using locum tenens physicians?

The 2009 survey suggests that the use of locum tenens physicians continues to be common among hospitals, medical groups, and government supported health care facilities. Nearly three quarters of health facility managers surveyed (72 percent) indicated that their facilities had used locum tenens physicians to supplement their existing medical staffs sometime during the last 12 months. This number is fairly consistent with the 77 percent who reported using locum tenens in 2007 and the 79 percent who reported using locum tenens in 2005. Staff Care's ongoing surveys indicate that the use of locum tenens physicians has now become the rule among most healthcare facilities rather than the exception.

Forty percent of those surveyed indicated that their facilities currently are seeking locum tenens physicians to supplement their existing medical staffs. This number declined relative to previous years tracked by the survey, in which at least 50 percent of facility managers surveyed indicated they were seeking locum tenens physicians. This decline may be a result of decreases in hospital and physician utilization brought on by the economic downturn, which also may have caused physicians to reduce their vacation times, increase their hours and take other steps that could inhibit the need for locum tenens physicians.

Over one-third of those surveyed (37 percent) indicated that in a "typical month" they do not use any locum tenens physicians. Locums tenens is either not part of this group's staffing strategy, or it remains only an occasional option. For the remaining 63 percent, however, locum tenens physicians are an ongoing resource. Forty-three percent of those surveyed indicated that they use at least four locum tenens physicians during a typical month, indicating that some facilities rely to a significant degree on the presence of temporary doctors. In 2007 and 2005, no more than seven percent of respondents said they use four or more locum tenens physicians in a typical month, suggesting that the gaps in medical staffs at certain facilities may have grown wider in recent years and are being filled with a growing number of locum tenens physicians.

The majority of those surveyed (56 percent) responded that finding locum tenens physicians is no more or less difficult today than it was 12 months ago. However, nearly one-third (30 percent) said that finding locum tenens physicians is more difficult today than it was 12 months ago, compared to 23 percent in 2007 and 20 percent in 2005. Fourteen percent said that finding locum tenens physicians is less difficult today than it was 12 months ago, compared to 16 percent in 2007 and 20 percent in 2005. That some facilities are finding it more difficult to find locum tenens physicians may be a result of the ongoing physician shortage (see below.)

Reasons for using locum tenens

Healthcare organizations use locum tenens physicians for a variety of reasons. The most common reason for using locum tenens referenced in the 2009 survey, cited by 37 percent of those interviewed, is to provide coverage for physicians on vacation or those pursuing continuing medical education. The second most common reason cited is to fill in until a permanent doctor is found. This response reflects an evolution in the locum tenens market that is linked to the national physician shortage. Historically, locum tenens doctors have been used to hold a place for ill, vacationing or otherwise absent doctors pending their return. Today, national doctor shortages have prompted hospitals, medical groups and others to use temporary doctors to maintain services in lieu of permanent doctors, who may be difficult to find.

In addition, the aging of the physician population (over one-third of physicians today are 55 years old or older) and the increased mobility of doctors can generate relatively high physician turnover rates at hospitals, medical groups and other facilities. According to the 2009 survey, 22 percent of health care facilities use locum tenens doctors to fill in for physicians who have left the area. Fourteen percent said they use locum tenens doctors to either help meet rising patient demand for medical services or to fill in during peak usage times such as flu season.

Interestingly, 25 percent of facilities managers surveyed said they use locum tenens physicians to test market new services, up from three percent in 2007 and four percent in 2005. By using a locum tenens physician, health facilities can determine whether their communities can support a new surgical, diagnostic or other medical service line, without the expense of hiring a full-time, permanent physician. An increasing number of facilities may be using locum tenens doctors in this strategic manner in order to better control costs during the current economic downturn.

The main benefit of using locum tenens physicians, cited by 36 percent of those surveyed, is to maintain continuity of patient care. However, by seeing patients who might otherwise have gone elsewhere, locum tenens physicians also allow medical facilities to maintain revenue streams. Twenty-three percent of those surveyed said that "preventing revenue loss" was a benefit of using locum tenens physicians. Using locum tenens physicians also can be part of a physician retention strategy. Sixteen percent of those surveyed cited "prevents existing staff burn-out" as a benefit of using locum tenens.

Surprisingly, 35 percent of those surveyed indicated that cost was one benefit of using locum tenens physicians, up from just 6 percent in 2007 and four percent in 2005. This may be attributable to the fact that more facility managers are determining that the cost of using locum tenens physicians can compare favorably in some cases to employing permanent physicians, when salaries, benefits and other expenses are considered.

How are locum tenens physicians perceived?

Healthcare facility managers were asked to rate the general skill level of locum tenens physicians. The majority (66 percent) rated locum tenens physicians' skills as either "good" or "excellent." Thirty-three percent rated their skills as "adequate", while a small number (1 percent) rated them as "unsatisfactory." The majority of respondents in 2007 (79 percent) also rated the skill level of locum tenens physicians are either "good" or "excellent." When locum tenens physicians first came into wide use, the quality of these physicians sometimes was questioned. Today, locum tenens practice has become more widely accepted by physicians, and physicians practicing locum tenens are rigorously screened. The 2009 survey suggests that quality concerns about locum tenens physicians have been largely put to rest.

Healthcare facility managers also were asked to indicate how locum tenens physicians are viewed by various parties, including permanent physicians on their staffs, the organization's administration, and patients. The majority (56 percent) said that locum tenens physicians are "accepted" by permanent staff physicians; 28 percent said they are "tolerated;" one percent said they are "not accepted;" and 16 percent were unsure. The majority (57 percent) said that locum tenens physicians are "accepted" by the administration; 25 percent said they are "tolerated;" two percent said they are "not accepted;" and 16 percent were unsure. Fifty-six percent said locum tenens physicians are "accepted" by patients; 13 percent said they are tolerated; zero percent said they were not accepted; and 31 percent said they were unsure.

In comparing locum tenens physicians to permanent physicians on their staffs, the majority of healthcare facility managers agreed that locum tenens physicians treat the same number of patients per day, spend the same amount of time with patients, and generate the same level of gross charges as permanent physicians.

Worth the cost?

Healthcare facilities pay a daily rate for the services of locum tenens physicians, a rate that can exceed $1,500, depending on the specialty. Balanced against this are the various benefits locum tenens doctors provide, including the ability to maintain both medical services and revenue. On balance, the majority of healthcare facility managers surveyed (79 percent) indicated that locum tenens physicians are worth the cost.

PART II

Survey of Physicians Working On A Locum Tenens Basis

Number of Providers Surveyed = 758

Key Findings:

The way physicians practice has been evolving rapidly over the last 10 to 15 years, as many doctors move away from the traditional full-time, private practice model to other modes of practice, including hospital employment, part-time practice, inpatient practice, concierge medicine and locum tenens.

Why do physicians choose to practice on a temporary basis? What are some of the characteristics of locum tenens physicians and to what extent do these physicians feel they are accepted by colleagues and patients?

Part II of Staff Care's 2009 Survey of Temporary Physician Staffing Trends, completed by physicians who work on a locum tenens basis, examines these and related questions.

Key findings include:

***Locum tenens physicians generally have multiple years of medical experience**.* 86 percent of locum tenens physicians surveyed indicated they have been in medical practice for 11 years or more. 67 percent have been in practice for 21 years or more.

Locum tenens continues to attract new physicians. 30 percent of those surveyed said they have one year or less of locum tenens experience, suggesting locum tenens continues to be embraced as a practice style by new physicians.

Most locum tenens physicians plan to stick with temporary practice. 63 percent of those surveyed said they plan to practice on a locum tenens basis for more than three years.

The majority of locum tenens physicians work six or fewer temporary assignments a year.
80 percent of locum tenens physicians work six or fewer temporary assignments a year.
53 percent work three or fewer such assignments per year.

Freedom trumps pay among locum tenens physicians. Freedom/flexibility was identified as a benefit of working locum tenens by 31 percent of those surveyed, compared to 15 who identified pay rate as a benefit.

The majority of locum tenens physicians feel accepted in the workplace. 96 percent of locum tenens physicians said they are accepted by patients, 86 percent said they are accepted by staff physicians, and 84 percent said they are accepted by facility administrators.

An analysis of these and other findings of Part II of the survey follows survey results below.

Part II: Questions Asked and Responses Received

1. What is your specialty?

Anesthesiology	17%
Behavioral Health	10%
Primary Care	20%
Radiology	22%
Surgery	16%
Other	15%

2. How many years have you been in medical practice?

	2009	2007	2005	2004
Less than 1 year	**2%**	5%	5%	n/a
1 to 5 years	**6%**	12%	9%	16%
6 to 10 years	**6%**	11%	10%	13%
11 to 20 years	**19%**	17%	22%	22%
21 or more years	**67%**	55%	54%	43%

3. How long have you worked as a locum tenens?

	2009	2007	2005	2004
Less than 1 year	**30%**	46%	33%	44%
1 to 3 years	**26%**	25%	31%	28%
More than 3 years	**49%**	29%	36%	28%

4. How long do you intend to work as a locum tenens?

2009

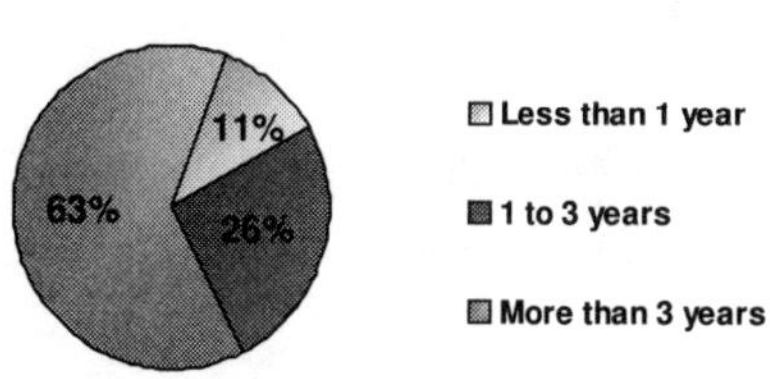

2007

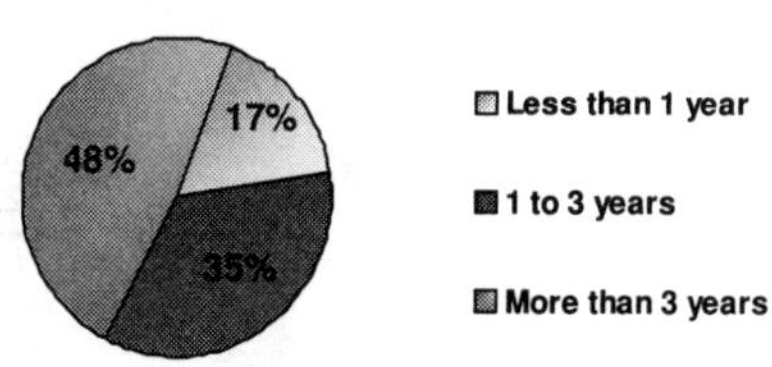

5. About how many locum tenens assignments do you work during a year?

	2009	2007	2005	2004
1 to 3	**53%**	60%	57%	55%
4 to 6	**27%**	24%	23%	34%
7 to 9	**10%**	4%	7%	6%
10 or more	**10%**	12%	13%	5%

6. What is your ideal locum tenens assignment length?

	2009	2007	2005	2004
Less than 1 month	**49%**	49%	35%	45%
1 to 4 months	**32%**	36%	50%	38%
5 to 8 months	**10%**	7%	11%	9%
9 to 12 months	**9%**	8%	4%	8%

7. Have you ever worked in a permanent position?

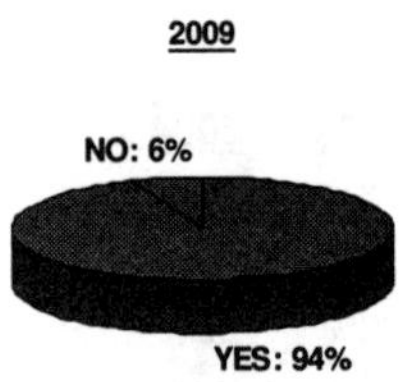

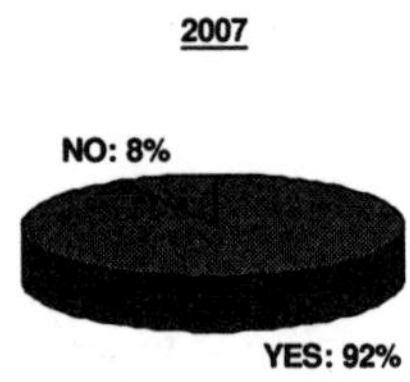

8. If yes, how would you rate working as a locum tenens versus working in a permanent position?

	2009	2007	2005
Locum tenens is MORE satisfying	**16%**	19%	62%
Locum tenens is LESS satisfying	**21%**	14%	20%
Both types are EQUALLY satisfying	**63%**	67%	18%

9. Are you currently looking for a permanent position?

	2009	2007	2005	2004
Yes	**23%**	23%	22%	22%
No	**77%**	77%	78%	78%

10. What are the benefits/drawbacks of working as a locum tenens?

Benefits	2007	2007	2005
Freedom/ flexibility	**31%**	79%	85%
No politics	**19%**	45%	44%
Travel	**18%**	44%	46%
Pay rate	**15%**	42%	38%
Professional development	**9%**	27%	27%
A way to find perm	**7%**	19%	19%

Drawbacks	2009	2007	2005
Away from home	**31%**	61%	63%
Uncertainty of assignment	**25%**	52%	47%
Lack of benefits	**17%**	33%	44%
Quality of assignment	**13%**	18%	25%
Other	**2%**	14%	9%

11. With how many locum tenens agencies do you work?

	2009	2007	2005	2004
None	**9%**	14%	6%	9%
1	**25%**	38%	31%	40%
2-3	**52%**	42%	50%	44%
4 or more	**14%**	6%	13%	7%

12. How do you select a firm?

	2009	2007	2005	2004
Location of opportunities	**20%**	67%	60%	63%
Customer service	**22%**	51%	57%	45%
Pay rate	**16%**	50%	47%	49%
Reputation/name recognition	**14%**	34%	42%	28%
Number of opportunities	**16%**	34%	39%	28%
Malpractice insurance	**10%**	26%	32%	21%
Other	**1%**	12%	11%	15%

13. How do you select temporary opportunities?

	2009	2007	2005	2004
Location	**23%**	86%	83%	84%
Pay	**13%**	58%	55%	55%
Length of opportunity	**29%**	57%	61%	45%
Type/size of facility	**7%**	28%	32%	28%
Quality of Equipment	**4%**	23%	10%	n/a
Patient load	**8%**	22%	35%	15%
Available shifts	**15%**	n/a	n/a	n/a

14. How far are you willing to travel?

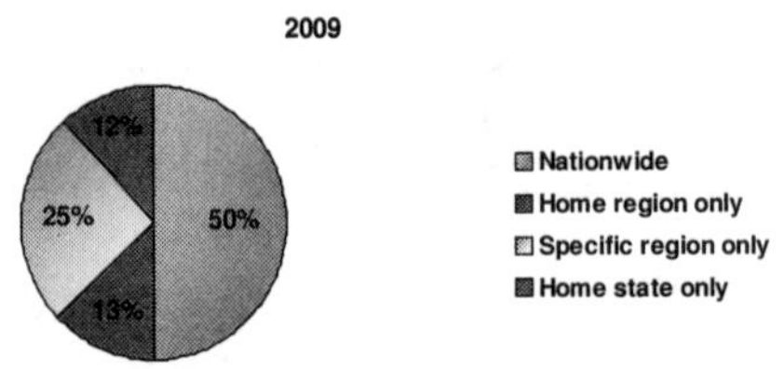

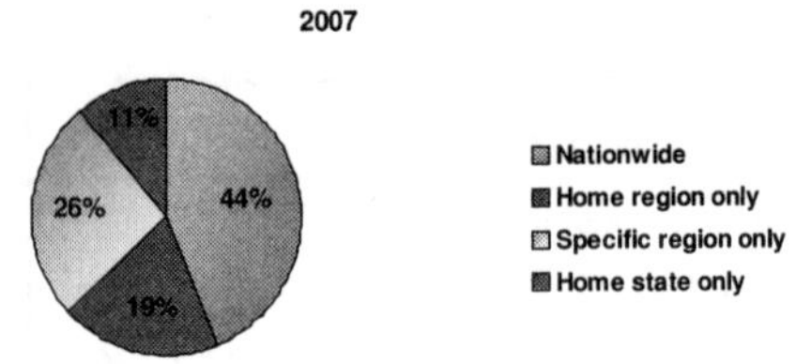

15. What value do you bring to a hiring facility?

	2009	2007	2005	2004
Maintain patient care	**33%**	90%	87%	56%
Prevent staff burnout	**22%**	52%	56%	8%
Generate revenue	**23%**	46%	52%	15%
Add a specific skill	**19%**	39%	40%	n/a
Uncertain	**n/a**	n/a	n/a	14%
Other 3	**n/a**	n/a	n/a	7%

16. As a locum tenens provider, how do you feel you are viewed by…?

2009

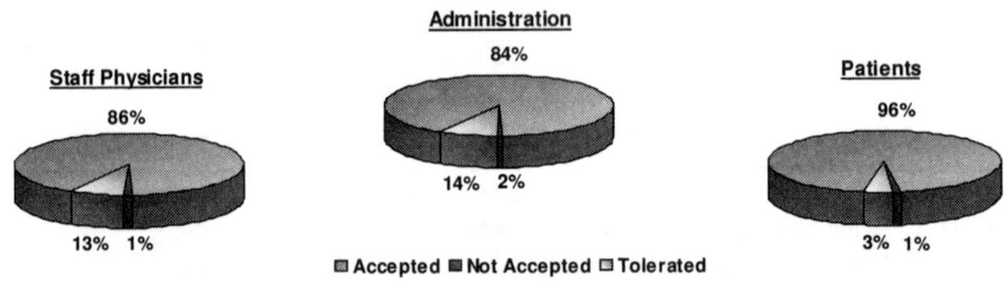

2007

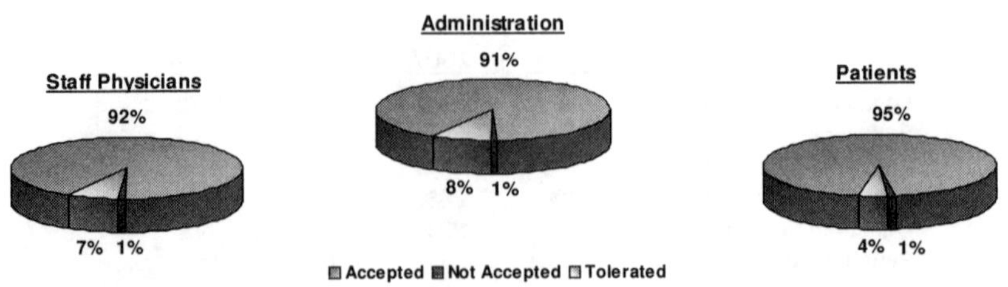

Trends and Observations

Part II of Staff Care's 2009 Survey of Temporary Physician Staffing Trends reflects several characteristics of locum tenens physicians and suggests some of the reasons why they work on a temporary basis.

Who are locum tenens physicians?

Over two-thirds of locum tenens physicians surveyed (67 percent) have 21 years or more experience as physicians. By contrast, some of those surveyed are relatively new to medicine. Seven percent have been in practice five years or less, while 25 percent have been in practice from six to 20 years. The 2009 Survey therefore indicates that locum tenens physicians vary widely in terms of medical practice experience, though the majority are highly experienced physicians who have been in medicine for two decades or longer.

While many of those surveyed have considerable experience as physicians, about one third are relatively new to locum tenens practice. Thirty percent have worked locum tenens for less than one year, while 26 percent have between one and three years of locum tenens experience. Forty-nine percent of those surveyed may be classified as "veterans" who have three or more years experience working as locum tenens. As in previous surveys, the 2009 Review indicates that a significant number of locum tenens doctors are relatively new to temporary medical practice and that the ranks of locum tenens doctors continue to be replenished and expanded by physicians who are newly attracted to the field.

The majority of physicians surveyed (53 percent) work one to three locum tenens assignments per year. About one quarter (27%) work four to six assignments, while 20 percent work seven or more assignments. These numbers suggest that some locum tenens physicians are also in permanent practice and "moonlight" on temporary assignments during vacation time or other opportunities. These physicians may only work a limited number of locum tenens assignments each year, while other physicians who are not in permanent practice may work temporary assignments on multiple occasions or even throughout the year. Other physicians, while working only two or three temporary assignments a year, may work on longer assignments that, combined, can take up a significant portion of the calendar year.

Forty-nine percent of physicians surveyed said their ideal temporary assignment length is less than one month, which reflects the fact that many locum tenens physicians have limited windows during which they can work temporary assignments. Thirty-two percent indicated their ideal assignment length was one to four months, while 19 percent preferred assignment lengths of five months or longer, demonstrating that some locum tenens doctors work temporary assignments on virtually a full-time basis.

The survey indicates that many physicians view locum tenens as a long-term career option. About two-thirds (63 percent) indicated they plan to practice on a temporary basis for more than three years. Another 26 percent plan to work locums for an intermediate length of time (from one to three years) while the minority (11 percent) said they will practice locums for one year or less. This indicates that some doctors use locum tenens as a short-term option that serves as a transition to another stage in their careers, while others make it a lasting career choice.

Ninety-four percent of physicians surveyed have worked in a permanent position, while six percent have worked only locum tenens. Of those who have worked in a permanent position, 63 percent indicated that permanent medical work and temporary work are "equally satisfying", while 16 percent rate locum tenens work as "more satisfying" than permanent and 21 percent rate permanent positions as "more satisfying" than temporary.

Why practice locums?

When asked why they practice locum tenens, 31 percent of those surveyed identified "flexible schedule" as a reason, followed by 19 percent who cited "no politics" and 18 percent who cited "travel." By contrast, only 15 percent cited "pay rate" as a reason for working locum tenens. For most physicians, locum tenens represents a lifestyle choice and not necessarily a chance to enhance their incomes. Locum tenens also represents an opportunity to escape medical politics and the other so-called "hassle factors" of traditional medicine, such as having to pay high premiums for malpractice insurance, which is typically provided for them by staffing agencies such as Staff Care.

Being away from family and friends was the most frequently cited drawback to locum tenens practice, referenced by 31 percent of those surveyed, followed by "uncertainty of assignments," cited by 25 percent. In some cases, locum tenens physicians are unable to schedule assignments as continuously as they would prefer. "Lack of benefits" was a drawback cited by 17 percent of those surveyed. This reflects the fact that locum tenens physicians are independent contractors and are not employed by temporary staffing agencies. They may get certain benefits through their permanent employers as they "moonlight" on temporary assignments or they may arrange for their own health insurance and other benefits.

The majority of those surveyed (91 percent) work with at least one temporary staffing company, while 66 percent work with at least two. Though they do not employ physicians, temporary physician staffing companies help match them with opportunities and arrange for many of the logistics, such as travel and accommodations, and often assist with licensure and credentialing. Twenty percent of physicians surveyed select staffing firms based on the practice locations offered, while 22 percent select firms based on the customer service provided. Pay rate, name recognition of the firm, and number of opportunities offered also were among the most frequently listed reasons for selecting particular staffing agencies.

When asked how they select a temporary opportunity, 29 percent of physicians surveyed identified "length of assignment" as a factor, followed by 23 percent who identified "location" and 15 percent who identified "available shifts." Thirteen percent identified "pay" as a factor contributing to their decision to select a particular opportunity. As independent contractors, locum tenens physicians are able to select which locations they prefer as well as what level of pay they wish to accept. If a particular staffing firm is not able to match them with a location they prefer, they may choose to work through another firm or contract directly with a hospital or medical group.

What value do they bring?

When asked what value they bring to a medical facility, 33 percent of locum tenens physicians surveyed identified "maintaining patient care" as a key factor, followed by "generating revenue" (52 percent). Twenty-two percent indicated that they help facilities to "avoid staff burn-out" while 19 percent indicated they add a clinical skill.

Locum tenens physicians were asked to what degree they are accepted by other physicians, administrators and patients. Locum tenens physicians have been a part of the medical landscape for some 30 years and the survey indicates they have become generally accepted. The great majority of locum tenens physicians interviewed (86 percent) indicated they are accepted by permanent physicians with whom they work at their temporary assignments, while 96 percent said they are accepted by patients, and 84 percent said they were accepted by administrators.

As the use of locum tenens physicians has become more common, and as privileging requirements and practices have become more stringent, concerns that may have existed about the quality of care provided by locum tenens physicians appear to be fading.

PART III

Review of Staff Care's 2008 Temporary Physician Staffing Assignments

In the course of a calendar year, Staff Care conducts thousands of temporary physician search assignments for its clients, seeking to match independent contractor physicians in multiple specialties with hospitals, medical groups, government facilities and other organizations requiring the services of *locum tenens* physicians. Staff Care also conducts temporary staffing assignments for certified registered nurse anesthetists (CRNAs) and for dentists.

Following is a review of the temporary staffing assignments Staff Care conducted in calendar year 2008. The review reflects current trends in the locum tenens staffing industry, including which types of temporary healthcare providers are in particular demand.

Top Temporary Staffing Assignments By "Days Requested"

Staff Care tracks demand for temporary physician staffing services through the number of temporary physician "days requested" by its clients. The table below indicates the percentage of Staff Care's "days requested" in 2008 by medical specialty.

	2008	2007	2006
Primary Care	42.7%	41.5%	40.7%
Anesthesia (Anesthesiologists/ CRNAs)	20.2%	20%	22.4%
Behavioral Health	15.6%	17.6%	17.2%
Radiology	10.6%	11.6%	11.6%
Surgery	8.3%	7.7%	8.1%
Dentistry	2.6%	1.6%	N/A

Number of Days Filled, 2008 and 2007

In calendar year 2007, Staff Care filled 219,576 days of temporary assignments nationwide with locum tenens providers.

In calendar year 2008, Staff Care filled 222,340 days of temporary assignments nationwide with locum tenens providers.

Trends and Observations

The breakdown of temporary provider "days requested" above reflects current demand trends in locum tenens. "Days requested" indicates the number of temporary physician days in various specialties Staff Care was asked to fill by hospitals, medical groups and other healthcare facilities nationwide.

Primary care – including family practice, general internal medicine, and pediatrics – was the specialty area in greatest demand in 2008, as it was in 2007, with over twice the number of days requested of any other specialty area.

The rise in demand for locum tenens primary care physicians is symptomatic of a national shortage of these types of doctors. The shortage is a function of changing demographics, including both significant population growth and population aging, coupled with a stagnant to declining supply of primary care physicians. The Census Bureau projects that 50 million people will be added to the population between 2000 and 2020. This includes new births and millions of immigrants, many of whom are young and will require the services of family physicians and pediatricians. In addition, 75 million baby boomers will begin turning 65 and be eligible for Medicare in 2011. Older patients with multiple chronic conditions typically are treated by general internists. The supply of internists, however, is compromised by the fact that a growing number of internists are choosing to sub-specialize and are not entering primary care practice. A study appearing in the October, 2008 edition of the *Journal of the American Medical Association* indicates that only two percent of medical students plan to specialize in general internal medicine. The supply of family physicians is compromised by the fact that fewer U.S. medical school graduates are choosing to train in family medicine than have in the past. In 2007, 16 percent of family practice residency slots went unfilled, according to the Association of American Medical Colleges. Moreover, 52 percent of medical school graduates who elected to train in family practice in 2007 were international medical graduates, some of whom will return to their home countries after training.

As a result of these supply and demand trends, many hospitals and medical groups are unable to fill permanent positions for primary care doctors. Often, they use locum tenens physicians to maintain services and revenue until permanent positions can be filled, as is reflected in Part I of this Survey. This trend accelerated somewhat in primary care in 2008, which saw a slight increase in the number of temporary physician days requested over 2007.

By contrast, the economic downturn felt in 2008 and 2009 reduced utilization of healthcare services in some areas of the country, leading to fewer hospital admissions, fewer patient visits per physician and fewer procedures. As a result, physician days requested in anesthesia declined slightly from 2007 to 2008. A similar decline was seen in radiology which, in addition to the economic downturn, has been affected by changes in reimbursement that has constrained utilization in some areas.

Behavioral health is another area in which healthcare providers are in critically short supply. The Department of Health and Human Services projects that demand for general psychiatrists will increase 19 percent between 1995 and 2020, while demand for child and adolescent psychiatry will increase by 100 percent during the same period. Meanwhile, the number of psychiatrists being trained is projected to remain static at best. In many cases, behavioral health facilities, particularly state funded institutions and correctional facilities, already cannot find psychiatrists to fill permanent positions and are dependant on locum tenens providers to maintain services.

However, behavioral health also is often poorly funded, and such funds that exist frequently are reduced during economic slowdowns when state and other monies for behavioral health can be cut. In addition, rising unemployment and the loss of health insurance that goes with it can decrease patient ability to pay for behavioral health services. These trends may be reflected in the slight decrease in behavioral health days requested from 2007 to 2008.

Demand for surgical locum tenens services has remained steady over the last three years, as tracked by Staff Care's Survey. Within surgical fields, demand is particularly strong for general surgeons, who often are referred to as the "primary care providers" of surgery because their services are less specialized and often less well remunerated than services provided by other surgical specialists. Like primary care physicians, general surgeons are in great demand and short supply. The lack of general surgeons and other types of surgeons in certain geographic areas has kept demand for locum tenens surgeons at a consistent level over the last three years.

Locum tenens has been an established tradition in medicine for many years but is still a relatively new concept in dentistry. However, as the number of dental schools and dental school graduates in the U.S. has remained fixed in recent years, while the population has grown rapidly, a shortage of dentists is emerging that is driving the use of locum tenens practitioners. Several years ago, Staff Care received virtually no requests for locum tenens dentists. Today, the firm receives thousands of such requests from state-supported and private dental practices nationwide.

For more information about this survey, please contact:

Staff Care®
An AMN Healthcare Company

5001 Statesman Drive
Irving, Texas 75063
800-685-2272
www.staffcare.com

Proud Sponsor:

Country Doctor of the Year®

104{

NOTES

106{

Staff Care®

An AMN Healthcare Company

5001 Statesman Drive
Irving, Texas 75063
800-685-2272
www.staffcare.com

Proud Sponsor:

COUNTRY DOCTOR OF THE YEAR®

ABOUT STAFF CARE AND AMN HEALTHCARE}

Established in 1992, Staff Care is the largest locum tenens staffing firm in the United States, placing physicians, certified registered nurse anesthetists (CRNAs) and other clinical professionals on temporary assignments nationwide. As an AMN Healthcare company, Staff Care is part of the largest healthcare staffing organization in the country. The entire family of AMN Healthcare companies follows:

BRAND	CATEGORY	QUICK RESPONSE *4-8 Weeks*	TRAVEL *13-26 Weeks*	LONG-TERM *9-12 Months*	PERMANENT PLACEMENT
Staff Care	Physician	X	X	X	
Merritt Hawkins & Associates	Physician				X
American Mobile Healthcare	Nurse		X		
Nurse Choice	Nurse	X			
Medical Express	Nurse		X		
NursesRX	Nurse		X		
O'Grady Peyton International	Nurse			X	X
Med Travelers	Allied	X	X		
Platinum Select Staffing	Allied	X	X		
RxPro Health	Allied	X			X

For additional information about the contents of this book, or to inquire about Staff Care's services, webinars and speaking presentations, please contact:

STAFF CARE
An AMN Healthcare Company
5001 Statesman Drive
Irving, TX 75063

(800) 685-2272
(469) 524-1473

StaffCare.com
AMNHealthcare.com